The Medicalization of Cyk

C000172739

The entire infrastructure and culture of medicine are being transformed by digital technology, the Internet and mobile devices. Cyberspace is now regularly used to provide medical advice and medication, with great numbers of sufferers immersing themselves within virtual communities. What are the implications of this medicalization of cyberspace for how people make sense of health and identity?

The Medicalization of Cyberspace is the first book to explore the relationship between digital culture, medical sociology and bioethics. It examines how technology is redefining expectations of and relationships with medical culture, and addresses the following questions:

- How will the rise of digital communities affect traditional notions of medical expertise?
- What will the medicalization of cyberspace mean in a new era of posthuman enhancements?
- How should we regard hype and exaggeration about science in the media and how can this encourage public engagement with bioethics?

This book looks at the complex interactions between health, medicalization, cyberculture, the body and identity. It addresses topical issues, such as medical governance, reproductive rights, eating disorders, Web 2.0 and perspectives on posthumanism. It is essential reading for health care professionals and social, philosophical and cultural theorists of health.

Andy Miah is Reader in New Media and Bioethics at the University of the West of Scotland and a Fellow of the Institute for Ethics and Emerging Technologies, USA.

Emma Rich is Lecturer in Gender, Identity and Health at Loughborough University, UK.

The Medicalization of Cyberspace

Andy Miah and Emma Rich

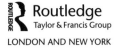

LONDON AND NEW YORK

First published 2008 by Routledge
2 Park Square, Milton Park, Abingdon, Oxon OX14 4RN

Simultaneously published in the USA and Canada
by Routledge
270 Madison Avenue, New York, NY 10016

Routledge is an imprint of the Taylor & Francis Group, an informa business

Typeset in Times by
GreenGate Publishing Services, Tonbridge, Kent

Printed and bound in Great Britain by
TJ International, Padstow, Cornwall

British Library Cataloguing in Publication Data
A catalogue record for this book is available from the British Library

Library of Congress Cataloging in Publication Data
Miah, Andy, 1975-
 The medicalization of cyberspace / Andy Miah and Emma Rich.
   p. cm.
 Includes bibliographical references and index.
 ISBN 978-0-415-37622-8 (hardcover) -- ISBN 978-0-415-39364-5 (pbk.) --
ISBN 978-0-203-93113-4 (electronic bk.) 1. Medical telematics. 2. Medical
informatics. 3. Social medicine. I. Rich, Emma, 1977- II. Title.
 R119.95.M53 2008
 025.06'61--dc22

                              2007033707

ISBN 10: 0-415-37622-X (hbk)
ISBN 10: 0-415-39364-7 (pbk)
ISBN 10: 0-203-93113-0 (ebk)

ISBN 13: 978-0-415-37622-8 (hbk)
ISBN 13: 978-0-415-39364-5 (pbk)
ISBN 13: 978-0-203-93113-4 (ebk)

For our families
Para nuestras familias

Contents

Preface

In the early 1990s, a number of guides to the Internet were published in hard copy, which aimed to introduce the World Wide Web to new users. It is not our intention to provide any such guide in relation to health or medicine. Today, the printed Internet guide is already redundant, and the best place to begin any searches will always be online. In our view, medicalized cyberspace emerges of its own volition and can, at times, stand in contrast to the need for official guides to anything. Nevertheless, the notion of guidance interests us greatly, and this text is concerned with the increasing range of health resources that are found within digital environments like the Internet. In particular, we respond to the emergence of non-regulated health information online, which became a challenge to institutions that saw their capacity to organize health information challenged by the decentralized character of the Internet.

Our medicalized cyberspace is also unconcerned by the idea that types of online behaviour should provoke medical concern, as indicated by Quinn (2001). We are not interested in Internet addiction or any such behavioural aspects of using digital technologies. Nevertheless, the language through which such ideas have been conveyed is pertinent to our analysis. Moreover, these observations are integral to the symbolic associations that arise in relation to rhetorics about the Internet (e.g. technophobia or, conversely, addiction).

Instead, our ideas for this book connect with our claim that there is something originary about the Internet in shaping knowledge, culture and society. Moreover, we argue that cyberspaces are critical components in fashioning cultural products associated with health and medicine. However, if it could be said that our work is some kind of a guide, it is more of a historical navigation than an explanation of how to find specific material online. Additionally, the book does not describe *cultures* of cybermedicalization, since we have not developed a typology of communities and practices. Again, we also suggest that such claims misconstrue the ways in which mobility and loyalty to particular spaces operate online. Nevertheless, there exists a medicalized cyberspace that is characterized by the notion of *becoming*, which is constituted by a process of negotiations of and around body and health issues. This fascination has guided our approach to defining e-health or cybermedicine as the various formal and informal performances of health-related issues within a digital terrain.

Our argument raises questions for those who might seek such a guide and urges the consideration of how the Web and its technologies evolve. We seek to cultivate sensitivity towards digital culture's transitory form. Moreover, we claim that such sensitivity is what users grapple with as they negotiate new medical terrain in cyberspace, which emerges and changes almost on a daily basis.

This book has also developed out of other research themes. We have both written about the intersections of health *in* culture, though mostly in quite different contexts. Yet for both of us our works have become embroiled within arguments about medicalization, which are implied by claims about the legitimate ends of medical treatment and the notion of a biocultural – rather than biomedical – model of health. While discussions about medicalization have been visible in a range of contemporary studies, the literature on the emergence of health phenomena in cyberspace, particularly within online and Internet environments, has often been segmented into distinct subject areas. For example, studies of medical sociology and the Internet, or, to use a phrase of Seale (2005), 'critical internet health studies', are often completely separate from studies of cyborgs (Haraway 1991). Also, conversations about medicalization have not really been discussed in the context of digital culture. One of our initial observations is that many of the current discussions around medicalization should be informed by what is taking place online, as the Internet presents a crucial context where traditional, categorical assumptions about health, identity and medicine are being contested. For instance, the boundaries between patient and expert are blurred by cyberspace, where each category loses some aspect of its distinctive *modus operandi*. Alternatively, the medic faces new kinds of expectations and requirements in fulfilling the legal duty of care, and these require coming to terms with (Terry 1999).

The challenge of such confrontations to medicine is visible within a number of literatures that have identified the inadequacy of traditional assumptions about where medicine and health fit within society. For instance, the rise of debates on the public understanding of science is indicative of the problems provoked by the assumptions that are made by scientists and governments about the intellectual capacity of 'publics'. Today, few social scientists now write about the uninformed patient, or their need to be 'educated', although many governmental institutions still seem to treat their audience in this esteem. As such, a central aspect of scientific endeavour involves its communication, and a crucial mode of communication is now the Internet. In this context, a new era of collaborative medicine, of partnership health, of emerging alternative patient knowledges of health, renders medicalization a far more complex phenomenon than it previously has been. This also presents challenges for professionals who previously did not conceive of public engagement as part of their broader professional role. Yet it is also important to be cautious about what the Internet might provide. Too often, claims about digital culture are grounded in expectations of online emancipation for those who have been otherwise marginalized, or of having the capacity to offer an authoritative and legitimizing space through which quite marginal or radical ideas about the regulation of medicine can be made visible. We intend to probe the range of claims that can be made about digital cultures and to avoid such polarized and polemic expectations. While we consider that the Internet is enabling a range of important opportunities and challenges, we limit our claims about it being either a utopia or dystopia – and provide responses to those who would claim that it is either.

This book began in digital space during the summer of 2002 at the height of the dotcom crash and soon after the *BMJ* (formerly the *British Medical Journal*) published a series of papers on medicalization (Ebrahim 2002; Freemantle 2002; Melzer and Zimmern 2002; Moynihan and Smith 2002). At this time, one could foresee the enormous growth of online health services, and a literature was beginning to emerge about the role of informatics in medicine, notable from the publications within the *Journal of Medical Internet Research*. Yet there seemed to be almost no connections made between how digital technology might enable new kinds of medical practices and the theoretical work that had been undertaken by a range of cybercultural theorists who sought to, first, come to terms with what digital spaces meant to people. For instance, the works of such journals as *New Media and Society, Information, Communication and Society, Convergence* and *The Information Society* were absent from the regulatory debates that were taking place within medicine. Moreover, there was almost no discussion about the emergence of new kinds of platforms that were collectively described in 2005 by Tom O'Reilly as 'Web 2.0' environments, even though the spirit of such open spaces had existed for a few years. Nevertheless, around this time the Internet was beginning to change again.[1] Social software was beginning to change the ways in which people use the Internet, and this altered the character of Web-based communities. Social networking sites and other platforms that could facilitate collaboration and sharing between users brought an entirely different dimension to the notion of interactivity where large numbers of participants could contribute to the code that went into designing specific platforms. As a result, new kinds of online spaces began to emerge and new claims about the consequentiality of cyberspace were advanced. These new discourses on the Internet seemed to have rather more maturity than the early utopianism.

Our thesis developed in this context, as we endeavoured to piece together – and to some extent foresee the development of – these new assemblages of digital culture, where health was paramount. Very quickly, it became clear to us that a large part of the Internet's near future would be overlooked if one failed to consider the development of these new cyberspaces. For example, consider the attempt of Internet service providers in 2001 to eliminate Pro-Ana community websites, a case we shall discuss at length in Chapter 8. While reasonably successful at this time, the task became much harder in a Web 2.0 era, owing to the manner in which information became syndicated through RSS.[2]

Alongside these technological advances towards Web 2.0, the relevance of the concept of medicalization continues to be debated within various fields, made more complex by the recent social changes connected with postmodern agendas which have destabilized the authentic and authoritative position that particular health expertise was considered to have. As health discourse has become more diffuse, expertise has become subject to greater degrees of scepticism and critical reflection, as the application of authority within medical practice has been extended to many practices that are, for many, only dubiously health related. For example, alternative health care remedies, aesthetic surgical practices or, indeed, the over-treatment of health problems via pharmaceutical products such as Prozac, Viagra or Ritalin have often become characterized as lifestyle treatments, which involve different kinds of moral recognition (Elliott 2003). In this sense, the application of these technologies corresponds with the realm of pre-regulated, non-therapeutic, emerging medical interventions, which occupy an imagined social space not too distant from the tales found within science/medical fiction. In short, there has been considerable uncertainty over how medical ethics should deal with the prospect of lifestyle treatments. Accompanying this, a number of non-medical professionals have taken centre stage as experts on what is ethically acceptable within health care and medicine.

Early discourse around cyberspace and health drew upon a technologically determined articulation of cybermedicine and continued to imply some sort of moral hierarchy. While this was not typically seen as oppositional – and is increasingly being embraced by the professions – the manner in which the active medical non-expert is treated through professional discourses sustains the dominant role of the health care professional and the power relationship between patient and doctor specifically. This is demonstrated by the number of handbooks that are about navigating medical information online and the emphasis on reliability and regulation of information in cyberspace. The reliability discourse about cyberspace reveals how the Internet is framed by a presumption of a knowledge hierarchy. This is of concern, since its paternalistic character distracts from the reshaping of socio-medical relations that is taking place through virtual encounters. Uncertainty about whether cybermedicine could ever be comparable to non-cyber medicine (see Collste 2002) illustrates one of the founding scepticisms about cyberspace. It also presupposes that cybermedicine is necessarily less desirable than non-cyber medicine.

We claim that the scepticism over virtual medicine is largely unfounded and that cybermedicine can address a range of medicine's core concerns, such as the establishment of trust between patients and doctors. Yet, the implications of losing control of *medical information* are, for professions, tantamount to losing control of the profession itself. Evidence of this is offered when considering how online publishing has confronted various professions. During 2005–2006, the various discussions about Web 2.0 and blogging implied a shift in how authorship is made authoritative. Around this time, the first literary prizes to be given to bloggers spurred a number of reactions from publishing institutions, which promptly spoke about the importance of editorial decision making that would verify factual information and provide critical sources of judgement. In the context of health-related information, this kind of rhetoric also involves political force, and a good example of this concerns the regulation of online pharmacies, which will be discussed in Chapter 7. Within the rebordered Internet space, these problems are particularly difficult to manage. Indeed, if ever there are systems considered to be under threat by the decentralization of information, then it is those associated with medicine and health that seem to be among the most serious. To this extent, the most ardent worriers about the Internet's effect on society are those who envisage that it will lead to an anarchic dismantling of the established information systems and relationships that underpin medicine and health care. As Henson (1999: 373) expresses it, this could lead to greater prominence given to

> misleading or incorrect information by assuming that all sites are equal, by searching for only one or two sites at random or by searching for what they [patients] hope to be true. Information obtained from the Internet may conflict with recommendations provided by physicians, thus leading to confusion and uncertainty in the mind of the patient. The consequences of this uncertainty may lead to a delay in treatment or the patient turning to inappropriate forms of therapy.

This concern is intimately connected to the general priorities of medical ethics – an extension of a health care professional's duty of care, which is also integral to the information a patient receives and attempts to comprehend.

Much of what we argue rejects the idea that mixed zones of regulation will lead to greater confusion over medical information or that, if they do, this would be wholly problematic. Moreover, we consider that the decentralization of medical information is a positive step forward for how medicine is assumed (rather than consumed). In part, having too much information can provoke a greater reliance on engagement and the need to ask further questions about expert systems. The challenge ahead involves persuading policy makers to interpret the Internet rather than to treat it as a nuisance. Consequently, to situate these debates within the relevant broad cultural context, it will be useful to consider how studies of the Internet evolved, particularly in relation to issues of the body.

Many of the cases we draw upon in this book speak to specific instances of these debates. Discussions of this kind have also focused on the way cyberspatial diagnoses are changing the relationship between doctor and patient and the forms of health knowledge they generate. Indeed, cyberspace has also been the subject of moral panic concerning emerging phenomena. Numerous examples can be cited where the ways in which people are engaging with medicine are considered to be dangerous. For example, various misunderstandings are possible as a result of relying on a virtual consultant, who might badly advise a patient as a result of not having an informed appreciation of the individual's health. Earlier studies of health representations on the Internet were, therefore, preoccupied with the assessment of (medically defined) accuracy and quality (Seale 2005). This book approaches a broader conceptualization of medicalized cyberspace. We are interested in how various Internet communities construct health discourses and the sort of bioethical discussions that are being framed around particularly controversial cases online such as the pro-anorexic movement, reproductive technologies and the case of the auctioning of a kidney on eBay.

There are a number of complex reasons that might explain why Internet users seek out information about health and medicine. However, of particular interest to us is how digital space is being used as a means towards enriching communicative opportunities about medicine and how, in turn, this contributes to the redefining of health and medicine as a series of cultural practices and rituals. Importantly, these discourses transcend what might be more strictly aligned with health care policy issues, since many of the participants in digital medical tourism do not engage with the Web as a result of some illness they might have. For this reason, our analysis also provides an overview of ways in which cyberspace is appropriated within medical discourse, outlining the intriguing and diverse ways in which such expression is made manifest by new ways of writing text and representing selfhood. We consider that the contribution of the World Wide Web to a developed sense of social awareness and participatory culture is most noticeable from the way in which it has become a medium for medical or health-related information. These new cultural spaces encompass a range of social functions, from the established, authoritative and endorsed spaces of WebMD or portals for national health care systems, to the so-called dysfunctional cases of the Pro-AnaMia (anorexia/bulimia) sites, which consist of spaces where (young) people discuss their experiences of living with an eating disorder.

We are also interested in the way that cyberspace has become another media platform through which to govern health behaviour. We consider how cyberspace may feature in the 'endless series of health scares, backed up by government and public campaigns', which 'tend to encourage a sense of individual responsibility for disease' (Fitzpatrick 2001: 1). In this way, health phenomena enter the cultural arena via a negotiation of values. For example, when we began discussing ideas for this book, discourse was gathering rapid momentum around claims that western societies were in the midst of an obesity epidemic. Since then, a burgeoning body of research has highlighted how this discourse has translated into everyday practices imbued with moral imperatives to shape the body and one's lifestyle (Monaghan 2005; Rich and Evans 2005; Gard and Wright 2005). In terms of medicalization, obesity discourse is a powerful example of the recent expansion of medical authority into everyday environments. Moral imperatives connecting with weight regulation are ever-pervasive, impacting on virtually every social context, including cyberspace. Moreover, recent concerns over the phenomenon known as *size zero*[3] have recast eating disorders and slenderness back into popularist media debates. Increasing consumerism around health and weight online, coupled with the development of tools on the Internet for self-regulation of the body, are all emerging phenomena that reveal insights into processes of governance in cyberspace. While a literature exists on both of these matters, neither has explored fully the impact of cyberspace on these phenomena.

It is perhaps no surprise that the Web has given rise to a 'cultural turn' (Nash 2001) in medicine. As the great medium of our age, this cultural technology has enabled an engagement with medicine where the conventional spaces of home, leisure and work are conflated, offering an opportunity for home computing to redefine the professionalism of our everyday tasks. Previously, the use of computing indicated a sense of knowledge or expertise; today, that expertise has become domesticated. It is something that can be acquired with considerably more ease than has previously been the case. In short, the Web has provided a context for the development of alternative discourses of health. In this book, we explore some of these discourses, considering the transgressive bodies that are found in cyberspace and the construction of narratives of illness by non-health professionals. We consider that the way medical identity is reconstituted through the Internet reflects an emerging cultural politics of health, which disrupts and challenges established medical knowledge and the health care professions.[4] However, as we have noted, our approach to the medicalization of cyberspace is to see this as neither wholly liberatory nor disempowering. While much has been written about how cyberspace is challenging taken-for-granted assumptions about gender and sexuality, little has been revealed about how these concepts are mediated by a medicalization of the body. Yet cyberspace establishes even further evidence of how bodies are re-constituted via virtual spaces. By elucidating these links, we will gain a clearer understanding about the significance of digital technologies.

In sum, our expectations for this book are various. First, we offer this inquiry as a historical analysis of how cyberspace became medicalized and articulate this through various stories and critical moments in its definition. We explicate how cybermedicalization has shaped cyberspace itself and how it has changed biocultural features of other settings, such as the relationships between doctors and patients.

Second, we anticipate it being used by health care professionals as a resource through which to understand the complexity of virtual worlds and the communication of health. Cyberspace has been occupied by a number of health-related phenomena that have raised various complex and controversial ethical concerns. In exploring some of these contexts, we hope that our discussions may offer insight into the process of thinking through ethics within health-related professions. Moreover, we hope to encourage health care professionals to consider more fully how to embed digital spaces within their views about what constitutes modern medicine.

Third, we hope to contribute to the theoretical development of the medicalization thesis, particularly as it relates to Conrad (1992) and Illich (1975).

Finally, we intend to develop a transdisciplinary approach to understanding emerging technological cultures, particularly from a socio-cultural and applied ethical perspective. The growing prominence of ethical questions in cultural studies is an integral part of this interest and encompasses both Zylinksa's (2005) recognition of the need to relocate ethics, along with poststructural questions about the possibility of ethics in the context of an environment like the Internet. In short, the chapters in this book propose and explore a medicalization of cyberspace that involves the emergent practices, environments and phenomena that encourage medical sociologists, health professionals and ethicists to think about the distinction between virtual and non-virtual spaces.

Introduction

Medicine *in* society

In recent years, there has been a rapid expansion of health-related resources on the Internet and within other cyberspaces. In various medical discourses, it is widely recognized that these resources are used increasingly to access information about health, illness and medicine (Cook and Doyle 2002; Lewis 2006). Many articles that discuss how it is important for health care professionals to take into account the Internet begin with statistical citations about how many users are participating in this new cybermedical space. We will do the same. In 2006, it was reported by the Pew Internet & American Life Project 2006 that 80 per cent of all adult Internet users in the United States (over 113 million individuals) have searched for health information online (see Fox 2006). Indeed, health-related websites and discussion lists are said to be the most popular resources on the Web (Eaton 2002; Wilson 2002). Scholars of digital culture will not find this surprising. The prevalence of debates about the body and the Internet or virtual realities suggests that body issues are important subject matter to Internet users. To this extent, medicalized discourses on the body find a natural habitat within online environments.

Since Illich's (1975) early medicalization thesis, one can identify a critique of medicine that is framed by a concern about its encroachment into the social domain. The Internet has become one such domain where this medicalization is performed, or so we will argue. Within the United Kingdom, our country of residence, the value of the Internet to medicine was quickly subsumed within a discourse of patient empowerment that called for patients' active involvement in discussions about their health (Henwood *et al.* 2003). Moreover, the development of science communication and literature on the public engagement with science is constitutive of the breadth of research that is now investigating how to locate medicine *in* society, as has been true of research attempting to do the same with science (David 2005).

During the past five years, there have been numerous attempts to reconstitute this dynamic. In 2003, the influential think tank Demos reported on the potential use of mobile communication devices to transform health care in the United Kingdom (McCarthy and Miller 2003). Moreover, a number of new technologies are beginning to transform previously static assumptions about the isolatedness of being a patient. For instance, the development of emergency contact bracelets that can be pressed to call for help relocates vulnerable people via digital technology in quite profound and meaningful ways. These processes of redescription through technology recharacterize health – away from state and economic dependency towards communities of illness and the formation of an agency where health is consumed in an empowering manner. A broader feature of this recharacterization within an information-rich society has been the mediatization of health. In the sections that follow, we shall detail how health, illness and medicine have become features of disorderly discourses that are found within an increasing range of media.

Mediatized health

It has long been recognized that medicine has expanded its realm into the everyday, non-medical sphere, and a process of mediatization can be readily observed as a feature of this expansion. As Lyons (2000: 350) comments, 'previously, medical practitioners dominated coverage of health and illness information, whereas today there are a variety of voices to be heard, including dissident doctors, alternative therapists, journalists, campaigners, academics and so on'. Studies examining how health knowledge is constructed in various media continue to grow, examining newspapers (Coyle and Sykes 1998), magazines (Lyons and Willott 1999) and documentaries (Hodgetts and Chamberlain 1999, 2003; Lyons 2000). Our intention is to build upon the now well-rehearsed debates about the public's engagements with health and media and the impact these have on shared understandings of health. We are interested in how the mediatization of health is connected with discourses around aspects of disorderliness and its specific relationship with the Internet and the concomitant medicalization of cyberspace.

In this context, one should consider how the widespread concerns about obesity, eating disorders, cosmetic surgery, depression and smoking have entered the cultural arena as negotiations of value: the legitimacy of making 'bad' health choices versus the social interest in the healthy nation. The sorts of moral imperatives that can be seen within new public health promotion discourse (Peterson and Lupton 1996) are now a regular feature of contemporary media. An example of this is the film *Super Size Me* (Spurlock 2004), which sets out to dismantle the corporate foundation of (fast food) consumption. Its director, writer and presenter, Morgan Spurlock undertakes a thirty-day diet of nothing but McDonald's food. During this period, Spurlock's body becomes increasingly disordered – sick, fatigued and fat – and viewers are expected to observe the dangers of the fast food culture. *Super Size Me* is one of a host of health-related documentaries where the narrator uses their own body as an experiment through which to pursue a particular polemic, in this case the potential health risks associated with fast food culture. Other examples of cultural discourses on health include the Atkins diet and the many television programmes that attempt to deal with obesity in a range of ways – from seeming to assist and understand the lived experiences of people who are obese to the blatant objectification of them. Indeed, a recent movie on health care in the United States, *Sicko* (Moore 2007), from renowned protest director Michael Moore, illustrates the continuity of concern and prominence of these issues.

Also, there are a number of documentaries in the United Kingdom connected with the size zero phenomenon, where presenters undertake extreme dietary practices to demonstrate the risks associated with trying to achieve a US clothing size zero. Other shows have drawn upon the spectacle of the 'autobiographical' on display. For example, UK celebrity Ulrika Johnson's recent documentary *Am I a Sex Addict?* (Higham 2007) on sex addiction starts out as an investigative documentary but quickly takes a more personal focus when Ulrika finds herself questioning whether she too is a 'sex addict'. In these moments, the public are offered candid insights into Ulrika's private life as she undertakes therapy in front of the camera and deals with the medical diagnosis she is given. Similarly, in the United Kingdom in April 2007 the TV channel More4 (a Freeview channel owned by Channel 4) aired a series called *Shrink Rap,* which involves celebrities undergoing psychodynamic interviews and analysis with psychologist and former comedienne Pamela Stephenson. Biressi (2004: 335) suggests that such 'showcasing of personal trauma' can be seen in popular 'postdocumentary' culture such as 'TV talk shows, lifestyle programming and reality television'.

Controversial examples of the mediatization of bodily disorder include the Gunther von Hagens public autopsy and its subsequent television series *Autopsy,* which is part of his global interventions to bring autopsy closer to the non-dead public (Miah 2004). The public interest in what might now be described as the medical documentary (Dijck 2002) provides some insight into the growth of online film environments. Indeed, as the Internet becomes an increasingly sophisticated filmic environment, with the growth of platforms such as YouTube, the relationship between online resources and broadcasting becomes all the more meaningful and, perhaps, difficult.

Medicine in the media: 'do text in your body parts'

There are two aspects of television's relationship to the Internet that need to be considered in the context of our subject; these concern the casting of particular technologies as revelatory and the nature of expertise. One must understand the tendency of the documentary form to cast Internet technologies as 'futuristic' or 'revelatory', before explaining the character of medicalized cyberspace. Its promise of another-world is different from what is often articulated through medical documentary, which endeavours to normalize medical practice and verify its trustworthiness and legitimacy (Hodgetts and Chamberlain 1999). However, their common ground is found in the emergence of documentaries about future technologies, a sub-theme within the medical documentary genre rather than a complete break from it. These programmes are often difficult to construct, as there is rarely anything that can be filmed when the discussion is about technologies that do not yet exist or whose effects – or concept – are not yet known.[1] There have been clear instances where the medical and the cyber environments have met. For example, the chat show presenter and self-styled body adviser Vanessa

Feltz hosted the British television series *Cosmetic Surgery Live.* Her personality has been characterized through a staging of struggles with obesity, which, perhaps, serves to legitimize her credibility within such a programme. An integral part of this programme was audience engagement via mobile phone images. Viewers were encouraged to 'text in' their 'body parts', which could then be analysed by the programme's (American) cosmetic surgeon, either to suggest appropriate kinds of treatment or to dissuade people from considering such an intervention. This is one of the few instances where the sending of mobile phone images has been used within British television in this way.

While this instance fits within a range of programmes in which audience engagement via digital technologies becomes mundane, it contrasts with the manner in which the Internet is often treated as an alternative – sometimes, deviant – world, with its own laws, meanings and significances of which we should beware. There are numerous ways in which this fetish manifests itself, one of which is through news coverage that relies on the Internet as a resource. Frequently, television media treat the Internet as an authoritative space, where this act consolidates its authority, but which nevertheless brings specific pockets of webspace into the main 'stream' of information. We will discuss this occurrence later (see Chapter 6), in the context of the Ron's Angels website. Through these mediatized forms, authoritative discourses gain legitimacy in increasingly diverse ways. For example, one might consider how the imagery of the disordered body takes a central role in persuading the public of particular health risks. Indeed, mediatization often allows for the presentation of particular imagery, which can be considered part of a wider 'media spectacle' (Kellner 2003).

Cyberspace has expanded the range of authors who are able to produce spectacles of this kind. Moreover, it enables the rapid and vast circulation of such material. For example, in May 2007 a video of celebrity David Hasselhoff filmed privately by his daughter when he was drunk was made public via television and the Internet:

> David Hasselhoff asked his children to video him when drunk so he could 'see what he is like'. A video of the former Baywatch star, a recovering alcoholic, has now appeared on the internet, and shows him rolling around shirtless on a hotel room floor trying to eat a hamburger.
>
> (London Net 2007)

It is not difficult to appreciate how the mediatization of health is connected with discourses of the disordered body in occasions like these. The explicit spectacle of imagery and its moral narrative serves to problematize and medicalize particular behaviours, in this instance those connected with drinking and its relationship with alcoholism.

One might argue that mediatization may also enable the artistic expression of medical subjectivities, which can alleviate the often isolating circumstances in which sick people find themselves. A range of medical programmes in this genre testify to this in their capacity to convey the caring, though bloody and often dramatic, side of healthy disorder. Nevertheless, this has also raised challenges that have not yet found satisfactory resolutions. For example, the ability to ensure that consent is informed might be frustrated when the doctor is unable to see the circumstances under which a person orally agrees to something. Indeed, the process of communication can differ through a telephone compared with face-to-face contact. A further concern relates to broader processes of digitization within health care. For instance, DNA biobanks that would store information about research participants and patients have provoked concerns about the erosion of the public and private distinction, an issue that was raised first by the development of telemedicine (Bauer 2001). In part, these are the consequences of a broadening range of Internet participants, which have become an affront to the authority of health care professionals and the empowerment of patients. Yet they are also a reflection of the encroachment of the cultural political dimensions of health care provision into medical practice and its self-regulative authority. Scientists and physicians find themselves with the new burdens of communicating such complex notions of risk and science and engaging the patient's conviction of the Web's authority. The medicalization of cyberspace, again, challenges this established mode of communication. Alternatively, the broader representation of medicine within televised documentaries reinforces the legitimacy of medical expertise, and the inadequacy of a lay person's perspective (Hodgetts and Chamberlain 1999) becomes evident by the frequent absence of editorial control within online broadcasts or, at least, via the communicative variance of the video blog.

Health and medicine in cyberspace

Our arguments and claims derive from a number of theoretical observations on the prevalence of health-related discourses within society, and their manifestations within cyberspace. We draw from literature in cyberculture, which has been framed by questions of representation and subjectivity along with medical sociology to inform our analysis. Despite the existence of a wide range of literature in each of these areas, the relationship between cyberculture theory and cultural studies of health is still relatively underdeveloped. The expanding and ubiquitous presence of networked information raises ethical issues and challenges that connect to broader concerns around articulations of freedom of knowledge and with the current rearticulations of health outlined in the previous section. It is worth introducing here the wide range of health resources that are now available in cyberspace.

For many readers, some of these features may be familiar, as one only has to connect to the World Wide Web or open email to be exposed to advertisements about health products, medical devices or health services. These are not only imbued with health advice, but are often underpinned by a moral narrative about broader benefits. For example, Internet-based promotions for drugs such as Viagra – again, a case we shall discuss at length, in Chapter 7 – boast of their capacity to improve not only our health but also our lifestyles (Mamo and Fishman 2001).

Digitally enabled health services and cybermedicine are growing phenomena within the medical landscape, with the development of a range of services available on the Internet, including self-diagnosis information sites and online consultations with health professionals. The emergence of e-health and cybermedicine has therefore provoked a number of concerns: is it undermining belief in state-funded health care systems or, more significantly, revealing broader, fundamental inadequacies in relation to medicine and science? Conversely, can e-health be regarded as a form of alternative medicine? The medicalization of cyberspace has spawned a new lexicon for medical professionals, one that compels them to address how their communicative and professional stance might change as a result. As such, cyberspace raises questions about what constitutes biomedical knowledge and how technological cultures are central components in shaping medical discourses and knowledge economies. Many of these questions are framed by debates about whether the lack of regulation of Internet sites has the potential to translate into greater misunderstanding about health and medicine, rather than offering a greater opportunity to inform people (Burgermeister 2004). Questions of this sort first emerged with the development of telemedicine, which can be defined as the 'use of telecommunications and informational technologies to share and to maintain patient health information and to provide clinical care and health education to patients and professionals when distance separates the participants' (Field 1996: 27). Telemedicine has evolved into what is now recognized as cybermedicine. In general, it is useful to discuss cybermedicine as 'the science of applying Internet and global networking technologies to medicine and public health, of studying the impact and implications of the Internet, and of evaluating opportunities and the challenges for health care' (Eysenbach *et al.* 1999: 1–2). This book offers a critical account of the cultural politics of e-health attached to cybermedicine.

Initially, cybermedicine was seen as a challenge for the medical professions for its potential to transform the patient–doctor relationship, which would raise important regulatory questions about the ethics and practice of medicine (Pence 2000). For instance, Bauer (2004: 87) suggests that online physician–patient interactions will fail to achieve a suitable level of 'interconnectedness', thus interfering with 'the development of physician compassion and patient trust' (ibid.: 89). Bauer considers that this raises ethical issues, since it 'undermines the basic goal of medicine – the advancement of patient health and well-being' (ibid.). Alternatively, Collste (2002) notes that it is critical to understand how various examples of administering medicine via the Internet challenge conventional assumptions about the way in which a patient makes sense of their personal autonomy. So understood, the use of digital technology to perform health care assumes a specific kind of relationship between doctor and patient, which Collste (2002: 122) describes as the 'engineering-model':

> [O]ne can assume that the Internet consultation tends to resemble the engineering-model rather than a healing relationship. The consultation is made at

a distance and based on raw data, at least as long as the technical possibilities for IT-communication between doctor and patient are limited.

Conversely, the exponential growth of online resources has also been accompanied by considerable hype about the new capacities that e-health might bring. For example, the ease of accessing patients through digital networks could enable cybermedicine to offer even greater contact and 'bring a new egalitarianism to healthcare' (Makus 2001: 127) because of its capacity to bring about universal access.

In response, it seems (suspiciously) characteristic of expectations over the Internet that its collective influence is specifically as a tool either of *emancipation* or of *restriction*. Accordingly, the World Wide Web – or, more often than not, the specific search engine that is in favour – continues to be celebrated as a means of providing greater opportunities for the public to engage with medicine, and to understand the science of illness. This idea is reflected in studies that indicate how support is developed through sharing information and experiences of illness through chat-based online environments (Burrows *et al.* 2000). The opening of 'cyber-pharmacies' (Oliver 2000; Scaria 2003), WebMD, and the principles of cybermedicine more broadly, make possible the opportunity for non-medics to become more aware of their well-being and to find others who can provide information for them.

Our preferred use of the word 'cybermedicine' adopts an explicit stance towards a range of related discourses surrounding the use of digital technologies in the delivery of health care information and treatment. Telemedicine and more conventional concerns about medicine and the Internet tend to have focused upon pragmatic information management issues or matters relating to the doctor–patient relationship and the challenges posed by the virtualization of this relationship. In contrast, our use of cybermedicine considers in more depth the connections between medical sociology and cyberculture, as distinct from the phrases 'new media' or 'digital culture'. These latter phrases have, to some extent, broken from early studies on the prospects of the Internet, which imply some form of coming utopia. Indeed, if the post-1990 academic community of online researchers spent much of their time positioning their critical stance as denouncers of cyber-libertarianism, our positioning corresponds to a distancing from all revelatory expectations of the Internet – either as utopian or as dystopian. We seek neither to confirm nor to denounce these potentialities, nor even to project the Internet as a potentiality, which seems to be a term, curiously, aligned with only some kinds of technology. Rather, we are interested in the reasons that led to such great and grave expectations for this immense communicative structure that is the Internet. Nevertheless, it will be necessary to track the historical development of these expectations as they, too, reveal something about the frame surrounding the relationship between medicine and the Internet.

One might describe the wide range of issues pertaining to cybermedicine we consider as broadly matters of social justice or ethics – our attempt to relocate

ethics within cultural studies (Zylinska 2005). Thus, worries about dysfunctional online medical communities, the diminished trustworthiness of
information systems, or greater or lesser access to, and flexibility of, health
care and distributed information systems provoke ethical concerns within the
medical profession. It is not our intention to simplify or valorize the relationship between cyberspace and health. To some extent, we see the medicalization
of cyberspace as analogous to a novel medical discovery – not quite a cure for
cancer, but, in this trope, an artefact on to which profound expectations and
imaginations are placed. In the process, our text attempts to foster some critical
reflections on these processes and the complex array of outcomes they make
manifest. Our formal response to these claims about the prospects of a cyber-
utopia is explained through the concept of posthumanism, which we will also
define here. Posthumanism is a critical construct for making sense of the kind
of medicalization to which we refer. It encompasses a number of key ideological concepts that we seek to problematize. Posthumanism also extends the
cyborgian critique of humanity, arguing that moving beyond humanness does
not rely solely (or wholly) upon high technology or human–machine integration. Rather, the core implications of posthumanism relate to its redefinition of
ideology and the relationship between nature and technology.

In response to the early questions about the suitability of telephonic practices for medicine, our own position is similarly unforgiving and cautious about
the developments of cybermedicine, though this should not be construed as a
lack of enthusiasm for technological innovation. Rather, we suggest that some
of the worries that have been articulated about the medicalization of cyberspace
and, indeed, the virtualization of medicine are intimately connected to cultural
discourses on the machinic and its capacity to dehumanize society in broad
terms. Indeed, precisely these narratives emerge in relation to 'Rudy the Robot
Doctor', launched by the University of California Davis medical centre
(Dobson 2004). While Rudy was not an autonomous robot, it enabled a physician to come face to face with a patient when they were not in the same physical
location. The physician could guide the robot through the hospital ward and,
through it, could talk with people along the way. Yet an important piece of
rhetoric ensues when a story like this is broken. For, clearly, Rudy is neither a
robot nor a doctor, but more of a hybrid entity. It makes no sense to give Rudy
an identity, which, of course, is invoked by its being given a name and a physical, seemingly autonomous, presence that closely resembles the traditional
humanoid robot form seen in countless science fiction films. It is this type of
example that should be kept in mind as we approach our exploration of posthumanism in Chapter 9.

We also identify the interplay of power relations associated with the
rearrangement of medical information through the Internet. We have little doubt
that this interplay is oriented around forms of consumption, but we will suggest
that the means of production are also an integral part of the emerging cyber-
landscape. This justifies making the distinction between cyber- and
telemedicine and arguing on behalf of the former as the distinct mode of virtual

medicine. Yet Resnik (2001a) makes a further appeal to thinking about the prospects of cybermedicine. He describes a case where an earnest patient challenges the authority of his physician's diagnosis by bringing materials he has found on the Internet about his condition. Resnik (2001a: 148) notes that this challenge shapes the patient–doctor relationship in a way that leads to 'shared decisionmaking' rather than 'paternalism'. This challenge to medical ethics also resonates with our overall intention to explore how the democratization of knowledge through technology should temper fears about its being out of control.[2] However, we advance this thesis not without recognizing the challenges it raises, namely that the collapse of expert systems could also lead to greater vulnerability and a more impoverished health care system (Miah 2005).

Our project theorizes the medicalization of cyberspace by raising a number of issues and problems that have surrounded its development. We claim that cyberspace has become progressively medicalized and our intention is to examine this process in greater detail. In doing so we consider how cyberspace has been appropriated by a range of medical discourses, as they relate to social constructions of (ill) health. On this basis, we explore crucial shifts in wider understandings of health and medicalization through their constructions within cyberspace. To this extent, we do not assume that the medicalization of cyberspace merely sits within, or alongside, the medicalization of society; rather, we believe that it is culturally and sociologically distinct.

The Internet as a mass medium?

Throughout this text, we advance a claim about the increasing relevance of the Internet as an instrument of mass communication. To introduce this, we can consider the recent development of health care centres and practices where physicians have uploaded video clips to YouTube demonstrating specific treatments, such as how to use an inhaler for treating asthma. The expectation of such endeavours is, in part, that it will enable medics to reach a wider range of people than is possible to treat via their own practice. The performances bring crucial elements of personalised treatment, which are not easy to achieve via centralized policy initiatives. In particular, the bottom-up approach of online community support provides a democratized space, which benefits from the accumulated knowledge of *user-generated content*. Thus, the clinic's or doctor's performances enable patients to continue their personal relationship with their own doctor, through which there is an established degree of trust that might not be present in some comparable top-down initiative. This example illustrates the tension between centralized and decentralized information systems within the arena of medical expertise and how it challenges established ethical practices and principles. Embracing the latter of these systems involves confronting the prospect of an increasingly commercial and consumerist model of health that is deeply resisted by many aspects of the allied health care sciences.

The examples we use to inform our articulation of how cyberspace became medicalized cannot claim to be wholly representative of a generic community of users who are online, accessing medical or health-related information. Indeed, we consider that there are vast differences in how users access, utilize and interpret cyberspace as a provider of such information. Consequently, our interest in claiming that there is a general process of medicalizaton taking place within cyberspace requires that we say something about the digital divide. Indeed, where matters of health are concerned it seems particularly important to address the claim that access to online health care environments should be wide and diverse. It is important to address the divide, because it is one of the enduring challenges faced by those who argue on behalf of the Internet's capacity to bring about social change for the better. However, it is not our intention to explain how the Internet can become a solution for the major challenges faced by health care services, particularly those reliant on a state-funded scheme. Rather, we argue that it is important to consider the contribution that could be made by digital communication technologies to enrich health care services.

For many years, debates about the digital divide have drawn attention to how Internet access continues to be the domain of the privileged. These observations have raised questions about whether the Internet should be characterized as a mass medium at all. In part, this is because the channels of communication are more diverse than those for traditional media such as newspapers or television. However, it is also because audiences are much more fragmented and fickle in where they go for their information. In the era of the Internet, one tends not to think of a loyalty towards specific online information systems in the way that one might have talked about loyalty to television channels. Even the current domination of search engines such as Google can quickly be weakened as a more proficient system emerges. At most, one might characterize search engines as mechanisms of mass participation, but the character of information provision through online systems is different from the communicative act of television broadcasting or reporting. Importantly, users bookmark Google because they expect it to provide the best access to the desired information. It is neither simply information, nor a form of journalism.[3] Yet the immense waves of migration from one platform to another in cyberspace are tangible and the number of Internet users grows year upon year.

To the extent that there is now greater opportunity of access to the Internet, one might conclude that the digital divide is narrowing progressively, but in response to such a claim we would characterize the divide as much deeper than one relating to mere *access* to information. Rather, the division occurs at a more structural level. For even those who *do* have access to the Internet through their workplace, education, public services, mobile telephones and so on are not all members of online communities. As Wyatt *et al.* (2005: 213) note,

> Access involves much more than being in the vicinity of the right type of equipment: it also includes the gendered and generational social relations which form the context in which people's daily interactions or non-interactions with the internet take place.

Often, Internet usage performs very specific functions in people's lives, and it is not necessarily a regular leisure feature. To this extent, the Internet might not have the same meaning and value as more central communicative spaces and the social networks that surround them.

Our analysis begins by accepting that the digital divide is a perpetual but shifting nexus; it involves the possibility that expertise can dwindle, as, for instance, when a new PC operating system or browser technology requires the user to reskill.[4] By implication, it can also improve as platforms become more intuitive, which, we note, is a governing principle of many technological designs. Hence, we endeavour not to overlook claims that too much emphasis on the Internet overstates its role in delivering health care or any kind of service. Yet we also mention it in order to interrogate the designation of a space as 'cyber'. The move from analogue to digital offers considerable opportunities to propel non-Internet users into cyberspace, particularly as it allows the convergence of various kinds of technological systems.

We will make some suggestion that the divide is continually experiencing some degree of transformation, which at best indicates a narrowing, though at worst implies that a commercial model of Internet access still continues to structure and organize online behaviour. One might think of Rupert Murdoch's purchase of MySpace, Google's purchase of YouTube, or Yahoo!'s purchase of Flickr as indications of this shift. However, there are also instances of encouragement within public policy that are allowing more people to access more information for more of the time. For instance, some cities are beginning to treat wireless communications access as a public utility to be offered free by the city. This capacity is likely to grow with the introduction of more sophisticated wireless infrastructures and systems, such as WiMAX, which enable a vastly greater amount of information to be sent and received via a wireless connection.

Also, the convergence and diversification of handheld devices, including the pervasiveness of Internet-enabled mobile phones, would suggest that greater access is possible, even if many people do not yet use such devices for deep Web access.[5] It is also important to understand claims about the digital divide in the broader global context, which provide encouraging evidence of the narrowing divide. For example, over 480 million mobile phone users exist in China (People's Daily Online 2007), 17.0 million of whom use their phones to access the Web. As of January 2007, the total number of Internet users in China reached 137 million, and this figure is projected to overtake the number of users within the United States in just two years. In Beijing alone, there are nearly five million Internet users, 30.4 per cent of the city's population. Moreover, the proportion of Internet users in the under-30 age group has reached 72.1 per cent and the number of bloggers generally has reached 20.8 million (China Internet Network Information Center 2007; Weltao 2007). In all likelihood, the remaining population has limited access to a number of public or commercial services – cinemas, music, and so on – which indicates that there is nothing special about the digital divide, even if this does not diminish the importance of the divisions and the need to keep returning to issues of technological inequality.[6] In any case, the convergence of information platforms – mobiles, PCs, PDAs, and so on – challenges the particular arguments about the digital divide. Moreover, the emergence of Voice Over Internet Protocol (VOIP) is already transforming how people – admittedly, already wealthy people – consume voice data transmissions, increasingly as a free service. On this basis, it is not unreasonable to foresee a future where all voice communications become freely available, even if telecommunications companies find a way of charging customers for some other service. Indeed, this is already occurring, through the broadcasting of live television on handheld devices.

Many of the cases we will discuss have never reached mass or mainstream audiences, nor do they describe large communities. Thus, generalizability from our cases is not straightforward, nor should it be assumed that we claim to exhaust the range of medicalized cyberspaces that exist or, indeed, that have been important. In some cases, the strongest claim that we make would be to suggest that some of the examples we describe have been brought into the mainstream and mass public eye through their fetishization within traditional media. In many of our cases, the occurrence of a medicalized cyberspace has become the subject of controversy or moral panic – such as the auctioning of a kidney on eBay, or the emergence of Pro-Anorexia as a movement online, each of which we consider later. This moral panic over the digitization of real life will be relevant to our discussions about how officialdom positions itself within medicalized cyberspace.[7]

More broadly, generalization is an important issue to address, since theoretical work on the global society is also in transition because of the Internet. While the Internet is, in some sense, a global technology, there is no single, global entity of the Internet to speak of; it remains a disparate collection of stories, phenomena and experiences, which present the illusion of a global village but cannot be characterized in that way. A more suitable metaphor would be to talk of online communities as sets of global villages; types of micro-global space that do not map clearly on to the macro-global world. There are many trajectories along which medicalization takes place within and via these global villages.

Cyberspace may also be particularly symbolic of broader social developments, because its ontology derives from debates about the technological body: the cyborg, transhuman or posthuman. In this sense, the ethical issues that it presents are not confined to formal medical ethics, but encompass a more complex array of emerging issues which are less apparent within bioethics. Important questions emerge at this juncture; what medical discourses are appropriating cyberspace? How are subjectivities made available within and through medicalized spaces on the Internet? How is the increasing engagement with health issues online changing the nature of relationships between doctor and patient, or patient and health care? To this end, we explore how issues of medicalization, health and illness have been mediated by cyberspace. Such mediations offer new insights into, and understandings of, a number of health related phenomena.

By espousing a distinct thesis on digital culture, our intention is not to separate online from offline worlds. Nevertheless, a number of central issues confront our analysis. For example, we must ask whether the delivery of medical information should operate by different principles when it takes place online. We must also consider whether online spaces should be treated as environments, leisure spaces or even spaces of media production. Decisions about how such environments are classified influence the range of interpretations and assumptions for policy making one might make. Clearly, the Internet encompasses each of these types of space, though it is also distinct for its capacity to create novel spaces for which there is no regulatory precedent offered by established policies on the delivery of health care.

Overview of the text

To conclude this Introduction, we offer an overview of the book, to clarify our main arguments and points of analysis. Part I, 'Cybermedical discourse' draws upon key concepts within the fields of cyberculture, medical sociology and cultural studies. Chapter 1 provides an overview of the medicalization thesis, explaining how it relates to cyberspace.

Chapter 2 further contextualizes our theoretical parameters of cybermedicalization by reconsidering the implications of body studies of digital culture, as well as introducing some of the cybercultural literature we draw upon in our thesis. This chapter provides a digital culture retrospective within which we articulate our justifications for using particular kinds of terminology, in the context of the range of literatures that exist on cyber/web/digital/new media studies. We also explore the development of scholarly attention in this area, offering an initial indication of trends towards Web 2.0 and what this might signify for our analysis.

Chapter 3 gives an overview of the literature that has, thus far, been developed on the relationship between cybermedicalization and health expertise, particularly as it relates to issues of reliability and control.

In Chapter 4, we explain how cyberspace is now another context through which governance of health behaviour is achieved. We examine this within the context of a proliferation of online resources, which are utilized as technologies of self-regulation to prevent against obesity, including weight monitors, calorie counters and personal training services online. The emergence of these digital tools is situated within wider discourses that impart a moral imperative for individuals to assume responsibility for their health and to engage with an extensive self-surveillance of the body.

Chapter 5 extends our analysis of the complexity of competing discourses within cyberspace by examining patient narratives in cyberspace. With the emergence of home pages, blogs, and other Internet sources, cyberspace has been heralded as an unregulated context for people to (re)write their biographies in ways that may challenge biomedical discourses of health. We explore the complexities of this process by discussing how illness narratives associated with undiagnosed conditions encompass contradictory discourses around experiential and medicalized understandings of ill health. These narratives ground revelatory expectations of the Internet, illustrating that it is neither wholly utopian or dystopian.

Part II, 'Cybermedical bodies' outlines a number of cases of medicalized cyberspace that have spawned wider public debates and which have raised a number of complex questions about the substance of bioethical debates and the industry of bioethics. This second part of the book explains a number of cyber-medical moments that encompass the breadth of our broader thesis on medicalized cyberspace. Together, they represent the collapsing of boundaries between bodies and information, ethics and cultural studies, and the opposing political regimens of control and freedom, such as competing knowledge economies. The issues discussed in this second part of the book raise critical questions for those concerned with the governance of medical information over the Internet, or, perhaps, with the infiltration of medical space by non-regulated Internet entrepreneurs or communities. The title of Chapter 6, 'Partial prostitution', indicates our conclusion to that chapter, where we convey the idea that bodies and/as information are necessarily objectified and commercialized through online health encounters.

In the context of the shift from *identity tourism* to *body trafficking,* Chapter 7 notes that there is even greater concern about the inability to control (bodies within) virtual worlds. The concerns over partial prostitution give rise to discussions about what *biological property rights* one ought to have in cyberspace. We explore the common ground between intellectual and biological property before proposing that the medicalization of cyberspace constitutes a watershed for how we make sense of cyberspace and medicine.

Chapter 8 extends our interest in rights and regulation by examining Pro-Anorexia in cyberspace. This movement was created on the Internet (rather than in real time) and supports a 'managed approach to anorexia' (Fox *et al.* 2005b: 945), suggesting that an eating disorder can be a lifestyle choice. These cyber-spaces have often been produced and occupied by those who have experienced, or currently are experiencing, an eating disorder. Pro-Anorexia is a particularly interesting case from which to discuss emerging challenges of cybermedical spaces, since it is one of the few instances where servers have removed websites from the Internet.

Chapter 9 presents a posthuman reading of Pro-Anorexia communities and connects this with our wider thesis around the ethical challenges that the medicalization of cyberspace present. We consider how the medicalization of cyberspace urges us to reconsider the relationship between ethical and social scientific analysis of medical or pseudo-medical practices that stretch the limits of medicine's traditional goals. We also situate our arguments within various articulations of posthumanism, arguing that this concept helps focus our attention away from utopian or dystopian visions and towards the integrated cultural, political and media manifestations of debates about body modifications.

The conclusion completes our trajectory through the multifaceted and multi-disciplinary study of cybermedicine by attempting to articulate the role of ethics within such research. We consider how our investigation responds to evolving theoretical work that is interested in the relationship between information and bodies, along with the consideration that discourses on transhumanism are constitutive of a community resistive to the technologization of identity. Our response is to counter these concerns by drawing on the examples we have raised that call attention to the embodied practice of technologization – where trans- and posthuman rhetorics should be constructed as morally complex but not immoral. In doing so, we challenge the concern that biomedicalization needs to be construed as a dehumanizing process.

Part I
Cybermedical discourse

1 Medicalization *in* cyberspace

To appreciate what is involved in our examination of the medicalization of cyberspace, it is necessary to give a brief overview of some of its characteristics. We explore the various themes evident in the literature on medicalization, as they relate to cyberspace and offer some indication of the theoretical frame for our analysis. Our position is that an exploration of what is happening in online environments can gain from and contribute to wider theories on processes of medicalization. Medicalization is a widely used concept, and, for decades, it has been applied to an expansive range of literature across various fields, perhaps most notably within the sociology of health and illness (Broom and Woodward 1996; Ballard and Elston 2005). Tracing a detailed history of change in the way medicalization has been dealt with politically, academically and medically in the United Kingdom is beyond the scope of this book, though we do register some of the subtle shifts that have occurred in how it has been conceptualized in recent years. To that end, we highlight some of the key features of medicalization and the theoretical discussions that have ensued about the relevancy of this concept in contemporary society. Since our thesis on medicalization of cyberspace has its literary roots in Web studies, medical sociology, the sociology of health, and cyborgology, it provides a developing perspective on the concept of medicalization.

Medicalization and medical sociology

Studies in the area of health and illness, and medicalization, are numerous, and we take a broad view of the field's scope in this overview. The tendency for more and more problems to be treated as medical issues has long been of interest to sociologists, who have continued to recognize the effects of this process, referred to as medicalization. Since Illich (1975), the observation that medicine has found its way into more and more aspects of everyday life has featured in a range of writings across various disciplines exploring health and illness. Medicalization has become a guiding concept in exploring the processes 'by which non medical problems become defined and treated as medical problems, usually in terms of illnesses or disorders' (Conrad 1992: 209). Medical language now permeates many everyday activities, including childbirth, sex, reproduction, exercise, drinking, eating, smoking, and pregnancy, such that, as Komesaroff (1995: 21) observes, 'being a bit tired or irritable', which 'would most likely have once been put down to working too hard or having to put up with unpleasant social circumstances', now could provoke someone to 'see a psychotherapist or a naturopath'.

This process of medicalization has long captured the attention of medical sociologists, who have explored how these features of everyday life come to be viewed as diseases or medical conditions. A number of enduring critiques have been directed at the practices of diagnosing and labelling particular behaviour through medical discourse (see Illich 1975; Zola 1978; Conrad 1992). Zola states the issues directly:

> Medicine is becoming a major institution of social control, nudging aside, if not incorporating, the more traditional institutions of religion and law. It is becoming the new repository of truth, the place where absolute and often final judgments are made by supposedly morally neutral and objective experts. And these judgments are made, not in the name of virtue and legitimacy, but in the name of health. Moreover, this is not occurring through the political power physicians hold or can influence, but is largely an insidious and often undramatic phenomenon accomplished by 'medicalizing' much of the daily living, by making medicine and the labels 'healthy' and 'ill' relevant to an ever increasing part of human existence.
>
> (Zola 1998: 237)

Moreover, despite critiques (see also Broom and Woodward 1996; Lowenberg and Davis 1994) that highlight the potentially 'malign social consequences' (Komesaroff 1995: 2) of unwanted medical social control (see Zola 1972), medicalization is still rife within western culture.[1] Depending on which theoretical framework one employs, differing accounts of these processes of social control can be found. Contemporary reflections on medicine and society have, for decades, attempted to theorize this interdependent relationship, as succinctly captured in Komesaroff's (1995: 5) words: 'The technical outcomes of medicine and its conceptual forms may convey far-reaching social effects; conversely, the social forms find their expression in both medicine's theoretical structures and its practical techniques.'

Various theorists have also pointed out how the control of populations via medicalization tends to take place not via enforced action, but via the normalization of health behaviours within everyday contexts. Frequently cited in work of this kind, is Foucault's *The Birth of the Clinic* (1973), which has illustrated how various medical paradigms throughout history have provided a significant means through which we understand and experience our bodies and subjectivities. Medicalization has a significant impact upon these processes by introducing 'into previously unproblematic experiences evaluative discourse/meanings, evaluative criteria, which moreover, are presented as socially neutral, technical terms' (Komesaroff 1995: 4). This approach to health care is clearly evident within health promotion strategies oriented towards the prevention of ill health whereby

physical activity, alcohol consumption, diet, smoking, and body weight are subjected to a process of medicalization and everyday scrutiny. This kind of
'surveillance medicine' (Clarke and Olsen 1999: 23) renders an increasing number of everyday activities observable and treatable through medicine. Therefore, it
is suggested that medicalization may be shifting medicine from those who are ill,
to the lives of healthy people (Miles 1991: 183). This decisively impacts on the
meanings these activities have for many people, given that

> [w]e relate to ourselves and others, individually and collectively, through an
> ethic and in a form of life that is inextricably associated with medicine in all
> its incarnations. In this sense, medicine has done much more than define,
> diagnose and treat disease – it has helped make us the kinds of living crea-
> tures that we have become at the start of the 21st Century.
>
> (Rose 2007: 701)

Ethically, there are concerns that the practice of medicine is stretching beyond its
prescribed role and that this might diminish both the integrity of medicine and,
ultimately, patient care. One such case in which these arguments have arisen
concerns the medicalization of social behaviours. For example, what was previously considered as deviance might now be defined as medical disorder (see
Freidson 1975; Harwood 2006): 'What has been called crime, lunacy, degener-
acy, sin and even poverty is now being called illness, and social policy has been
moving toward adopting a perspective appropriate to the imputation of illness'
(Freidson 1975: 249). In this process, medical knowledge is constitutive in shifting 'badness' to 'sickness' (Conrad and Schneider 1980). Recent work by
Harwood (2006: 7) has provided compelling evidence of the effects of these
processes. On the basis of her critique of childhood behaviour disorder discourses, Harwood raises concerns that 'when a young person is diagnosed as
disorderly the diagnosis designates them as psychopathological. It is also likely
to signify that much of the child's behaviour, thoughts, even intentions can be
interpreted via the discourses of mental disorder'.

A number of other studies build on the above point by examining the effects
of medicalization upon the experiences and subjectivities of individuals. For
example, a growing body of work has examined the medical control of
women's bodies (see Miles 1991) through medicalization, and we shall explore
these issues further in Chapters 6 and 7. As Clarke and Olsen (1999: 3)
observe, 'gendered, cultured, historicised, classed, raced and otherwise situated, women are routinely silenced or erased as actors in the production of
health, in both the provision and receipt of health care per se as well as in
health politics and policy'. Similarly, Rose (2007: 369) argues that 'some
women are more medically made up than others – women more than men, the
wealthy differently from the poor, children more than adults, and of course, differently in different countries and regions of the world'. Subsequently, calls
have increasingly been made to 'revision – and thus to retheorize – women,
health and healing' (Clarke and Olsen, 1999: 3). While much has been written

about how cyberspace is challenging taken-for-granted assumptions about gender and sexuality, little has been revealed about how these concepts are mediated by a medicalization of the body. We explore a number of cases in Chapters 7, 8 and 9 that reveal the tendency for the Internet to provoke core feminist concerns about vulnerability and an ethics of care.

Issues of social control and medical power have, therefore, been central concerns in discussions on medicalization. Moreover, a number of problems arise in relation to the tendency to conflate the terms *medicalization* and *medical control*. Broom and Woodward (1996: 361) provide a useful distinction, suggesting that medical dominance

> is often a component of medicalization but is not identical with it. Medical dominance is evident in the conduct of consultations (when the doctors' priorities and views dictate what transpires) and in policy making (when the opinions and interests of doctors determine policy decisions) ... while medical dominance will often foster medicalization, the two are analytically distinct and may occur independently.

This is an important distinction to take into account when theorizing medicalization, since it affords the conceptual refinement necessary to make sense of the shifting and complex forms of social control that might or might not be present in differing forms of medicalization. Earlier theorizing of this term, while important in identifying the expansion of medicine into everyday lives, has since been subjected to a number of criticisms. Such critique was occasioned, in part, by the rapid expansion of social changes that earlier theories could not so adequately accommodate. Over the past two decades, the concept of medicalization has, thus, been a matter of significant discussion, and continual questions have arisen over its relevance to an increasingly complex society. In 2007, *The Lancet* published a series of papers (see Metzl and Herzig 2007) from a meeting in New York attended by interdisciplinary scholars 'seeking to address whether medicalization remains a viable notion in an age dominated by complex and often contradictory interactions between medicine, pharmaceutical companies and culture at large'. This collection of papers exemplifies the concerns that we raise about this concept and its ability to make sense of complex socio-medical phenomena. In particular, they address medicalization in so far as it implies the 'extension of medical authority beyond a legitimate boundary' (Rose 2007: 701).

Concerns have been voiced about the tendency within theories of medicalization to construct the lay public as passive. As Ballard and Elston (2005: 228) observe, 'earlier accounts of medicalization over-emphasized the medical profession's imperialistic tendencies and often underplayed the benefits of medicine'. Rose (2007: 701) urges caution over the tendency to imply that those who are medicalized are passive, arguing that 'although drug companies use techniques of modern marketing, they do not seek to dupe an essentially submissive audience'. Rather than being monolithic, these processes might be considered as 'multifaceted, multicomplex, in some places interlocking and in all cases involving relations of power, privilege, domination and subordination and always located within a specific cultural and his/herstorical context' (Clarke 1998: 47). Therefore, our interest is to consider how cyberspace provides a specific context within which various forms of medicalization may take place.

Consuming medicalization

Another approach to medicalization argues that it should not be attributed only to medical professionals. The role of consumerism, the expansion of health knowledge along with the positioning of 'pharmaceutical companies in the space once held by doctors as the supposed catalyst of social transformation' (Metzl and Herzig 2007: 697) have all influenced how medicalization takes place. The increased use of pharmaceutical products to combat particular conditions is now a feature of the contemporary health care industry. The Internet offers a unique contribution to these discussions; the emergence of online pharmacies is particularly visible in cyberspace. It has far-reaching consequences and has provoked responses from government, ethicists and health care institutions about the legitimacy of delivering products online and the often widespread condemnation of particular cases. Cyberspace offers a particularly rich context in which to explore some of these complexities of medicalization and commercialization. The worldwide distribution of pharmaceuticals – particularly those that have a non-therapeutic or 'lifestyle' function – crystallizes the challenges raised by the redrawing of boundaries that the Internet provokes (Moynihan *et al.* 2002). In Chapter 7, we connect processes of medicalization with online commerce, drawing upon the example of Viagra, which has been a visible and enduring component of discussions about online pharmacies. A range of conflicts of interest that are latent within the allied medical sciences and professions accompany these concerns. Thus, it is naïve to ignore the interest of pharmaceutical companies in supporting medicalization providing that it leads to the utilization of their products. Also, one must take into account the interests of health care services in seeking the most economically adequate solution to a particular problem, given the limitation of resources.

Other literature has revealed how 'medicalization is a much more complex, ambiguous, and contested process than the "medicalization thesis" of the 1970s implied' (Ballard and Elston, 2005: 228).[2] By alluding to a 'thoroughly medical form of life' that characterizes contemporary life, Rose (2007: 702) calls for a more critical evaluation of these heterogeneous developments. Each of these discussions can be informed by what is taking place online. Indeed, Conrad identifies that it is crucial to understand the 'impact of the Internet' (2005: 12) in constituting contemporary medicalization debates. Thus, while this book elucidates a process of medicalization of cyberspace, in doing so we suggest that this discussion should inform wider debates about the relevance of the concept of medicalization. Indeed, cyberspace is replete with unusual and emerging medicalized phenomena through which to expand the ethical discussion as to how, why and with what consequences differing forms of medicalization may occur. Therefore, cyberspace can provide an interesting case through which to expand on the concept of medicalization. This is important because certain complexities have been obscured through prior notions of medicalization.

> [t]he term medicalization obscures the differences between placing something under the sign of public health (as in the contemporary concern with childhood obesity), placing something under the authority of doctors to prescribe, even though not treating a disease (as in the dispensing of contraceptive pills to regulate normal fertility) and placing something within the field of molecular psychopharmacology (as in the prescription of drugs to alleviate feelings that would once have been aspects of everyday unhappiness).
>
> (Rose 2007: 701)

We are also interested in revealing subcultures of medicine on the Internet. We do so through our case studies, which reflect the intricacies and intimacies of medicalized cyberspace. In each of these cases, we explore the negotiations around medicalization taking place across various health/medical discourses.

In sum, despite continual critiques around medicalization, these ideas about the expansion of medicine into everyday life have remained influential, particularly in terms of the governance of medical knowledge. Indeed, public faith in biomedicine continues to remain strong (Lupton 1997). This also says something about the locus of control that governs scientific credibility, which is further disrupted by cyberspace. One of the central themes of our discussion about the medicalization of cyberspace concerns the relationship between ethical and social scientific analyses of medical or pseudo-medical practices that stretch the limits of medicine's traditional goals. Indeed, the phenomenon of medicalization itself can be characterized as an ethical issue, since it interrogates the legitimacy of professions through which trust and matters of personal privacy are invested. In Chapter 9, we make this ethical context explicit and offer explanations and responses to the positioning of ethics within medicalization work. Importantly, we do not presume that medicalization is inherently a damaging or negative phenomenon – or, at least, that no good comes from this characterization of particular behaviours and lifestyles. Our medicalization of cyberspace extends the work of these more recent explorations of medicalization by applying these ideas to the virtual reality of cyberspace. Our intention is not to give comprehensive ethical accounts of the manifestations of medicalization, but to highlight differing health discourses are made apparent in constructions of (ill) health and the body.

Throughout the text, we reveal how key trends within cybermedicine, such as the commercialization of body parts, patient-led support groups, or cyber-mediated illness stories, are altering both what are understood as the distinctions between biology and artifice (people and computers) and how we understand, construct, challenge or legitimize narratives of health and illness. To this end, our medicalization of cyberspace raises critical issues for bioethics, which might not be so readily expressed in other contexts. We hope that the insights from cyberspace will enhance an understanding of the complexity of the relationships between medical knowledge, discourse, society, identities and experiences of (ill) health. An interest in these issues is not new; however, they are raised here in the context of cyberspace with new dynamics and ethical features and, perhaps, differing impacts on people's experiences of health and the body. Crucially, the sort of ontological status we give to cyberspace has a bearing on the claims one might infer from health-related encounters. The crucial observation is that the claim that bodies are visible within cyberspace should not lead automatically to the claim that they are inscribed by sociological tropes. Underpinning each of these discussions is an interest in the relationship between medicine, medical knowledge and social context and values.

2   The cyborg body

In this chapter, we explore the theoretical parameters of cybermedicalization by considering the implications of body studies in digital culture. This analysis informs Part II, where we provide detailed cases of cybermedical bodies and develop the claim that the online body has always been gendered within cybercultural studies. It aims to establish a broad theoretical base through which to interpret medicalized cyberspaces.

Digital culture retrospective

In the early years of online research, identity politics emerged as a focal point for claims about how the Internet would reconfigure human relations. Scholars discussed its potential as a panacea for social injustice, a utopian space that would free people from the burdens that often emerge as a result of face-to-face interactions. Indeed, many authors often appeared to defend the view that the Internet would *not* enable this, though it was often unclear where any such view was asserted in the first place. Regardless, the claim was that these burdens encompassed the consequences of discriminatory judgements about one's body size, ethnicity, gender, age, and so on. The Internet was claimed to be a space where these body markers were absent and, thus, where one could inhabit cyberspace without the worries of being judged by these visible characteristics. Moreover, the claim recognized one's capacity to experiment with expressing one's identity by creating multiple personae within cyberspace (Donath 1996). Studies by such early cyber-libertarians as Rheingold (1993) cited instances of online emancipation experienced by those individuals who found themselves socially marginalised. These claims implied or dealt explicitly with a number of body concepts – such as gender, sexuality, ethnicity and age – and drew attention to the new possibilities for exploring identity within online environments.

Situating body metaphors in cyberspace was an ontological move that has framed the critical analyses of online interactions. Their invoking became part of the illusory architecture of the World Wide Web (Chesher 1997). For instance, if one takes the rhetoric of 'freedom' and 'constraint' that is both implied and explicit in some of the expectations present in the works of William Gibson (1984), John Perry Barlow (1996) and Howard Rheingold (1993), then one observes the significance of *embodied* space in cybercultural theory. Importantly, the Internet was conceived not merely as a free conceptual or communicative device, but as an *environment,* a location that enabled movement and exploration, where such terms as *surfing* and *browsing* became symbolic of what participation involved. Its cultural location was often discussed within the spheres of leisure (consumption) and, as Poster (1997: 216) states, the Internet was treated 'more like a social space than a thing so that its effects are more like those of Germany than those of hammers'.

These concepts implicate the body within cybercultures and involve a literal expectation where, as John Perry Barlow (1996) states, cyberspace is experienced as 'a world that all may enter without privilege or prejudice accorded by race, economic power, military force'.[1] The articulation of the Internet as a meaningful, communal world reinforces its corporeal status, which is visible within contemporary approaches to computing. As Tamblyn (1997: 42) notes, 'cyberspace is a manifestation of thought', and one can see a range of creative, expressive practices that it has spawned, from Net-Art to the Nintendo Wii. Moreover, these discussions arise within a broader context of inquiry that is interested in understanding how physical bodies fit within technological worlds.

The result has been an emphasis on understanding where the body is located within cyberspace, reflected by the vast number of investigations into representational issues that dominated early cybercultural studies. The conceptual basis for such inquiries is also extensive. For instance, the terminology used to describe computer-speak is often aligned with biological systems – for instance, one's files are vulnerable to *viral* infection – which extends this metaphorical relationship between human and computing systems. Indeed, this relationship is reinforced within the medical sphere, where technology often appears as a seamless part of the medical monitoring process.

Nevertheless, these claims by cyber-libertarians often involved little more than a simplistic (and mistaken) assumption that bodies are *absent* within cyberspace. Many scholars speculated that, just because people engage with each other through text-based communications, people would be free from the burdens of the body. Two important responses are necessary here. One has to do with our specific case: is the body really absent in cyberspace? The second has to do with the scholarly culture of *speculation,* which pervades cybercultural studies. We will address the latter of these issues later in the book, particularly in Chapter 9, but we wish to emphasize that the Internet appears to have become a speculative future-object for the scholarly community. By this we mean that the Internet occupies a space within scholarly research that is particularly interested in imagining the future.[2]

The belief that the body is absent in cyberspace was quickly informed by empirical studies that revealed a more complex set of circumstances. The body was not absent, but often re-presented in unfamiliar forms. Faced with the disappearance of the body in cyberspace, it became restated, written into the fabric of online encounters. Many forms of online interactions were based upon the performance of self-representation, and the mechanisms through which one did this were varied, but, critically, differed from face-to-face presentations. One difference was that the construction of a homepage[3] involved a process of imagining viewers that was qualitatively different from the processes in the inhabited space of the physical world, where the imagined audience is both present and visible. For instance, if one visits a nightclub, there is some reasonable basis on which to decide what kind of clothing would be suitable to wear. However, in cyberspace the form of self-presentation relies considerably on self-referential factors since there is an absence of well-defined social norms. For instance, if one perceives the Internet as a design space, an environment where aesthetic values are a priority, then greater care will be given to presenting a stylish image within a homepage. Alternatively, if one perceives it as a realist medium, then one might be more concerned with presenting all facets of one's persona, so the viewer can achieve a complete impression of one's character (Cheung 2004). However, these phenomena are often most visible in the websites of long-term Internet users or computer experts who strip their sites of any graphical content and make minimal use of variation in fonts, headings, and so on. These naked sites convey the priority of communication, accessibility and code. Of course, neither expectation is necessarily borne out in practice, since there is a considerable amount of slippage between design and reception.

In any case, the re-identification of the body in cyberspace brought with it a number of other claims about the significance of cyberspace, claims that sparked a polarization of views related to the Internet that has become an entrenched characteristic of media and cultural studies.[4] These positions might be crudely described as the techno-optimist and the techno-pessimist view, neither of which makes any specific claim about the value of technology. We mention the caveat because this dichotomy is often misconstrued. Thus, the techno-pessimist can be just as committed to the integration of technology in society as the techno-optimist. However, the pessimism perhaps conveys a doubt about the capacity to integrate these technologies into society in a way that offers a solution to entrenched social problems. The persistent concern about the digital divide is one clear example of this. We will see later how this polarization manifests itself in broader technological discourses.

Empirical studies of the Internet have sparked various kinds of divisions, most of which seem valuable and consistent with the emergence of any new subject area. For example, there are disputes about terminology: do we use the term 'cyberculture', 'Web studies', 'new media', 'digital cultural studies', and so on to define this area of inquiry? There have also been extensive debates about the ethics and methodology of online research, considering how it might be different from face-to-face data collection and what new ethical issues it might raise (Bassett and O'Riordan 2002; Ess 2002). Some of the decisions about the use of terminology are undisputed. For instance, to speak of a 'digital culture' in the 1990s would probably have been less meaningful than using the words 'Internet' or 'cyberculture', since the digital technology used by most individuals was limited to the Internet. Today, where digital communications have infiltrated a range of cultural and leisure domains, digital culture seems a more meaningful concept to describe academic research studies in this area. Alternatively, the word 'cyberculture' remains relevant for scholars within cultural anthropology, where 'Web studies' or 'new media studies' has emerged in, more, sociological studies on the Internet. Throughout our analysis, we rely on the notion of cyberculture. We do not think that it is yet possible to remove the *cyber* from studies of digital culture, as our claims imply something originary about the Internet in shaping contemporary culture. Thus, by utilizing the prefix *cyber* – which comes from the Greek, meaning 'to steer' – we suggest that cybercultural studies are also studies about how contemporary society is shaped by the emergence of many kinds of digital platforms.

In addition to these disciplinary differences, a more profound disagreement is latent within the broad range of cybercultural studies, which involves how researchers should treat online environments. The explanation of this position is found in Nakamura's (2002) notion of 'identity tourism', which she uses to describe how many of the early claims about online encounters referred to poorly (or mistakenly) conceptualized social spaces. Rather than freeing people from body burdens, experimentation with identity in online environments led to the further entrenching of stereotypes or, as she puts it, 'cybertypes': 'Rather than "honoring diversity" their performances online used race and gender as amusing prostheses to be donned and shed without "real life" consequences' (2002: 14).

However, the meaning one might derive from this observation is ambiguous. While we do not deny that meaningful understandings can emerge from studying, for instance, ethnicity within fiction, it is crucial to understand whether the attribution of a fictional character to an environment is appropriate. This is because it alters the kinds of claims we might make about the state of society – claims that are often advanced in relation to Internet youth culture. A helpful example that is closely connected to Nakamura's concern about ethnicity and our interest in claims about the consequences of unrealness is the 2007 British version of the reality television show *Celebrity Big Brother*, wherein a debate ensued about whether one of the participants behaved in a way that was racist. In this case, the discussions about the prevalence of racism in British society emerged in part because the actions of the individual involved – the self-styled celebrity famed for her participation in a previous non-celebrity *Big Brother*, Jade Goody – were subject to interpretation. Goody's actions sparked controversy, whereupon different interpretations of the programme were advanced. The crucial difference involved whether the racism expressed should be interpreted as the *intentional actions* of a particular individual (leading to an evaluation of the programme on the basis of standards of documentary) rather than the actions of a *staged performance* (which would involve its being treated as a form of light entertainment). While both types of activity have a similar capacity to yield something meaningful about what constitutes racism and, indeed, reveal something about the state of racism in society, the interpretation of the event itself differs vastly depending on which genre it is ascribed.[5] More succinctly, the entire episode would not have been headline news – and thus, the values of British society would not have been brought into question – if it had been a scripted drama, like a soap opera. Similarly, we suggest that the meanings and range of concerns that arise in the context of 'identity tourism' within the Internet depend significantly on what kind of 'tourism' is taking place.

We anticipate that Nakamura might not endorse our version of this term, since her derivation of it emerges from online phenomena that she describes as 'disturbing' (2002: 13). Yet this phrase also attributes an ambiguous ontological status to online environments, so it requires further interrogation. While Nakamura acknowledges the tendency for some academics to diminish the Internet as mere 'unreal' space, this claim is not unequivocal. Indeed, there are two aspects to the claim: one that we accept as mistaken and another, which is somewhat more ambiguous. Thus, it is mistaken to presume that these so-called unreal spaces are inconsequential; they are not simply playful or fictional. However, the degree to which online interactions can be treated as unambiguous social spaces is much less clear. Aycock (1993) describes how, 'in modernity, our experience of the real is primarily playful', suggesting a blurring of boundaries that is most noticeable in virtual communities. Consequently, the question arises as to what form of phenomenological experience might suitably describe the various types of online encounter when one is attempting to make identity claims.

Crucially, decisions about how online spaces are conceptualized have a bearing on the range of sociological claims one can make about them. For instance, do we treat the Internet domain as a social space or a creative space – not unreal or real, not fact or fantasy? A useful analogy might be to consider a drama class within which explorations of identity, values and the legitimacy of specific modes of communication take place. In this case, we can study the relationships within the class sociologically, but our claims about what we find are located in assumptions about what drama classes entail, as spaces of expressive creation, where people put themselves into specific modes of behaviour in order to explore their values, and so on. Clearly, the Internet is a collection of various types of space, and we might only suppose that this becomes more intriguing and complex as such entities as the game environment Second Life emerge. For example, in 2007 the Swedish government located an embassy within Second Life, and other realspace institutions have set up buildings and held meetings within this graphical two-dimensional environment. This adds even further complexity to our attempt to conceptualize such environments in sociological terms.

Nevertheless, for our present purposes the crucial observation is that the claim that bodies are visible within cyberspace should not lead automatically to the assumption that they are inscribed with the same sociological tropes as one might apply outside of cyberspace. In some sense, these performances might best be treated as scripted, wherein our task as ethnographers is the analysis of the text, rather than the society. We offer this argument not to diminish the importance of such spaces, but to temper the claims that one can infer unambiguously, from online behaviour, something about the state of society.

To a large extent, this framework for conceptualizing computer-mediated communications as unreal or future spaces remains dominant in the literature. Its implied relegation to the domain of speculation is reflected by how many chapters on the Internet within cultural studies texts are found at the end of the book, thus confirming the status of the Internet as a futuristic construct. We find this perfectly justified in one important theoretical sense, though this is often not articulated: the Internet remains a transitory epistemological domain, where semiotic or sociologic claims are framed by uncertainty, owing to the relative infancy of the Internet's historical trajectory. As some indication of this, one only has to identify the number of studies that identify various eras of the Internet, such as that by Mainzer (1998). While academics like to believe that their observations are eyewitness accounts of society in transition, the various claims about Internet transitions have often been relatively inconsequential to the intimate communities of Web developers.

The scholarly fascination with claiming that new eras are ushered in by, say, the possibility of connecting through wireless fidelity (wi-fi), or the pervasiveness of mobile media more generally, is often challenged by an unfairly named conservatism. More generously, such views are fundamentally worried about, for instance, how wi-fi might accentuate social concerns, such as pervasive surveillance, which could limit individual freedoms rather than extend them. To this extent, they should be (and are) taken quite seriously. Over the past few years, an additional claim to some form of 'new era' might be claimed in the context of 'Web 2.0', notably a phrase not defined by academics but one that emerges from within the practice community of online entrepreneurs (*see* Wikipedia 2007). Examples of online tools that make this visibility possible include a range of social software, such as Wikipedia, Flickr, YouTube, Frappr, Facebook, MySpace and others. These facilities made redundant many of the previous limitations on people's access to information online. Even the exploratory language used to describe Web activity is less integral to the parlance of online users. Today, people talk less about *homepages* and more about *presence,* marking a decentralizing of individual identity through syndication tools such as *technorati.*

While the distinct meaning of the concept is disputed, Web 2.0 designates a transition towards a set of structures that has transformed online publishing. Moreover, it has given rise to stronger claims about the capacity for online communication to enable activism or for it to be a mechanism for advancing citizenship. These new innovations make the earlier Web – Web 1.0, one presumes – look considerably limited. For instance, in the era of Web 2.0, many of the online publishing platforms no longer require a user to purchase software or, indeed, to have many more skills than the ability to navigate a website and follow onscreen instructions. Integral to this has been the rise of Web logging (blogging), which, for many people, persuasively democratizes online publishing compared to web publishing more generally, but which also appears to successfully disrupt the information hierarchy of the Web. For example, if one considers how websites become ranked within a search engine like Google – or indeed others – important differences have occurred. In the early years of the twenty-first century, search engines would continue to sell access to improved ranking. Today, one's capacity to attain high ranking relies significantly on *knowledge* about the most effective tools through which one can climb the Google ranking. To this extent, information – medical or otherwise – is even further reconstituted by an individual's capacity to negotiate visibility, often over and above the capacity of established institutions.

Importantly, many of these elements of Web 2.0 are ephemeral by design. For instance, many blogs now allow users to export their entire blog content to another service provider by means of a couple of clicks, thus allowing users to move freely between preferred platforms. Yet the significance of impermanence is also different in cyberspace.[6] For example, one might consider how intellectual property rights (IPR) are temporarily made unintelligible by online publication. If one publishes online some form of material that could be claimed to be a breach of copyright, then it is likely that the host site will be required to remove it after a period of time. Indeed, it is possible that users will notify the host about this breach, in the same way that users' flagging of inappropriate material establishes the moral culture of a Web 2.0 platform. Yet the removal of this copyrighted material will not occur until after a critical period of time during which the impact of the information is at its height. To this extent, the inability to assert IPR rapidly makes them partially inconsequential.[7]

These recent transformations of the Internet also provide further responses to the theoretical debates about *community* that pervaded cybercultural studies in the late 1990s (e.g. Clayton 1997; Holmes 1997; Jones 1995, 1997a, b). The nomadic communities within social software platforms such as Facebook or Second Life have reconstituted expectations about community identities within cyberspace, where there seems greater strength in using the term to describe one's Web presence. Debates about the realness of these environments are also all but over. Nevertheless, it is useful to remember that these aspirations for Internet users, to achieve the status of communities, represent ideals, continual works in progress, which are fragile and easily destroyed. These thoughts reinforce the similarities between online and offline social spaces and the challenges they face.

Perhaps a useful place to conclude this retrospective is in relation to discussions over *credibility,* a concern to which we continually return in the context of medicalization. The lack of 'realness' attributed to cyberspace brought with it questions over the trustfulness of people's actions, and intentions, and the dissemination of information. It is only recently that the Web has begun to provide robust responses to the challenge of credibility, though it is important to recognize that Web users are more sophisticated today, and in the same way that one might not worry too much that people believe everything they read in the newspapers or see on the television, there is reason to believe that methods of discerning reliable information online are also sophisticated. Indeed, the emergence of Google Scholar brings the prospect of completely reconstituting the debate about credibility (Giustini 2005). Also, the rise of open-access journal publications brings the possibility of transforming the relationship between scholars and readers and, in so doing, transforming the information hierarchies that underpin the current system of dissemination. Online search tools are now almost indistinguishable from library search tools and so the quality issues are less significant.

These changes to the ontological foundations of the Web – from text to textual; from *developer* designed to *user* designed – present a moment of crisis for online sociology. This crisis is visible in the emerging shift towards a fascination with studying mobile communications.[8] Identities have, once again, become a visible part of our (cyber) culture. Social software rejects the *identity play* of anonymity and the overwhelming attention by research inquiries into representation. Furthermore, the presumed fragmented presence of netizens is becoming increasingly joined together through really simple syndication (RSS). Moreover, there is greater recognition that legitimacy of opinion is afforded by participation in cybersociety. Many of the online environments are practices that require some degree of immersion before it becomes clear what range of capacities they facilitate.

The presence of a medicalized body within cyberspace has been visible since these early Internet studies. However, more broadly, our thesis develops in the context of literature on cyborgs, which has been an integral part of many cybercultural studies. The broad range of cyborg technologies that have been discussed over the past fifteen years function across two, overlapping, communities of scholarly interest. The first involves the notion of disability and reparation of the sick body via technology. The latter augments the body through artistic practices and ritual. Importantly, each of these contexts blurs with discussions about the capacity of cyborg technologies to usher in what might be described as a world of posthumanity, a concept that we will return to later. Here, we want to discuss the various themes of cyborgology and how they relate to cyberbodies.

The *cyber* part of the terms 'cyborg' (in full, cybernetic organism) and 'cyberculture' are often unhelpfully conflated within the literature. While Nayar (2004) makes explicit the connections between -borgs and -cultures, there are important distinctions. As Devoss (2000: 838–839) notes,

> The term 'cyber' refers to a term coined much earlier [than Haraway's 'cyborg'], but popularized by William Gibson, a popular science fiction writer, in his 1984 book, *Neuromancer*. Cyberbodies are 'high-tech' bodies that, instead of problematizing representations of bodies and the heterosexual imperative in much visual representation, reproduce norms of sexuality and the sexualization of certain women's bodies, and validate the male gaze. The cyberbody does not politicize the potential of the techno/synthetic/mechanical body in the ways that theorized notions of cyborg bodies can.

It is relevant to discuss the implications of this conflation, though we wish to explain it as a conceptual lens, a mechanism for propagating the medicalized body in cyberspace. In this manner, we describe the conflation as a form of *cyborg ritual,* the components of which are revealed in a much wider survey of ideas.

The cyborg ritual

Haraway's 'Cyborg Manifesto' has become the cornerstone of inquiries into understanding the political claims associated with technological transformations of the body. Her work on cyborgs originates as a text concerned particularly with mythologizing a 'post-gender world' (Haraway 1991: 150). Similarly, Braidotti

(2002: 241) argues that 'the body in the cyborg model is neither physical nor mechanical – nor is it only textual'. Its digital humanness has little to do with the process of immortalization as argued through interpretations on the Visible Human Project (VHP), or rendering more visible the human (Waldby 1997, 2000a). More accurately, it is an Invisible Human Project (iVHP) concerned with the project of eternal youth (Springer 1996).

Yet how widespread has the influence of Haraway's cyborgology been on discussions about medical technology, as opposed to, say, science fiction literature on the same concept? We advance the idea that the function of the cyborg has been largely *ritualistic,* rather than literal, or explanatory of human–machine interactions. The cyborg is invoked not simply as a symbolic metaphor, but as a performance, recurrent and varied rather than merely represented and invoked. Numerous examples of such performative cyborg rituals exist, though it is important to draw attention to examples that might not immediately feature as cyborg performances. For example, the film *The Fly* (Cronenberg 1986) employs various articulations of the cyborg, though there is no physical interfacing of machine and human. In this case, while the cyborg narrative relies on the *prospect* of teleportation – the reduction of matter into particles and their subsequent reconstitution – its more substantive cyborgian gesture is its representation of transgenics: what happens when the genes of different species are mixed. In this context, *The Fly* is particularly interesting, since the act of mixing genes is shown to be a human oversight, as opposed to the frequent depiction of seemingly good science that simply goes wrong.[9] Certainly, the scientific intention within *The Fly* did go wrong, but what went wrong never had any bearing on what was originally intended. Had the intent actually been to mix genes, then this kind of mistake would have been more straightforward.

The overlap between the narrative within *The Fly* and contemporary scientific developments becomes constitutive of the ethical concern and the objectionable character of the cyborg. Yet while the mistake depicted in *The Fly* is *unequivocal,* the mistake of xenotransplantation is only *prospective;* it engages the possibility that the mixing of species could give rise to some weakening of humanity's distinctiveness, or a risk to its existence. Moreover, the fly itself signifies the single unit of complexity – the cell; its minuscule size is impossible to anticipate or observe, not unlike the course of biological transformation. Thus, *The Fly* warns of the complexity of science and the challenge of controlling for molecular-sized variations. *The Fly* explains how the cyborg ritual has become an integral part of cultural texts, and how their presence within artistic expressions have both constituted imaginations about the prospects of science and become the sole signifier of the signified cyborg. Within media discourses, this ritualistic practice of affirming the morality of cyborg cultures is embedded within many kinds of reportage.

The work of this cyborg ritual needs further contextualization within other artistic endeavours and, by revealing these broader conceptual connections, we begin to understand how discussions about the control of medical information online are situated within other cultural political processes. For example, discussions about the unreality of virtual worlds are correlative with the cultural locale of fictive texts. Each is regarded as a lesser, or deviant, sphere of concern compared with society or the proper realm of medical practice and, yet, they are both integral aspects of cyberculture's past, where popularized examples of such ideas in film include *The Matrix* (Wachowski and Wachowski 1999), *The Lawnmower Man* (Leonard 1992) and *Johnny Mnemonic* (Longo 1995). Additionally, the *bodies* (of work) of such artists as Stelarc or Orlan have become uncritically affirmative of the cyborg's elevated social status. Yet while these depictions of the cyborg engage the sociological imagination in quite novel ways, they do not wholly correspond with what Haraway intended when introducing the term. Thus, Haraway (1988) argues for 'situated knowledges' and is interested in the 'cyborg mundane' (Peterson 2007) as much as (or perhaps more than) its radical potential. Yet public engagement with 'infomedicine' (Thacker 1998) necessarily stems from what Waldby (1997) considers to be a popular anxiety and fascination for the potential of medical technologies. In part, this is what is intriguing about medicalized cyberspaces. Digital environments prompt us to reflect upon how we theorize and understand such concepts as embodiment. Whereas the body interfaces with technology, embodiment extends beyond the physical and visceral.

These interpretations should provoke suspicion over cyborg ritualization, when it is used to conceptualize new technological cultures. Yet it should also explain why we are stuck with the concept, in a similar way to how Turney (1998) describes our being stuck with Mary Shelley's *Frankenstein* text as a metaphor for bad science. Our task is to accept that discourses of panic will arise and to ask what should follow from their occurrence – in short, to transcend the polarized positions of bioliberalism and bioconservatism. In the context of cybermedicalization, we argue that, precisely because we are speaking of an interactive context – Web communities – the application of a Frankensteinian narrative is less appropriate; though paradoxically, it is also more prevalent.

Since Haraway's (1991) 'manifesto for cyborgs', concepts such as hybrid and cyborg now dissolve traditional boundaries around nature/culture and subject/object, and around what it means to be human. We take up some of the challenges posed by cyberspace in relation to the theorizing of humanness, which implores us to reconsider how

> [t]he human organism is neither wholly human, nor just an organism. It is an abstraction machine, which captures, transforms and produces interconnections. The power of such an organism is certainly neither constrained by nor confined to consciousness.
>
> (Braidotti 2002: 226)

Medicalizing the human through cyberspace makes humanness redundant as a defining characteristic of identity. Instead, such concepts as avatars, personhood, prosthesis and competence have become more useful articulations of differences. In part, this explains the recent development of studies that utilize posthumanism to refer to these contested concepts or, perhaps, the inadequacy of new ideas (i.e. post-isms generally and the cyborg, or transhuman, in particular).[10]

In response to this, we have attempted to reset the terms by which posthuman encounters are currently framed, by asking what questions arise subsequent to the polarization of bioconservatism and bioliberalism. The cyborg ritual reiterates the entrenched divide between nature and nurture that is visible within the contemporary clash between sociology and the post-genomic world of synthetic biology. As Braidotti (2002: 228) indicates,

> The spaces in between what is between the human and the machines, that is to say a dense materiality, post-human bodies are also surprisingly generative, in that they stubbornly and relentlessly reproduce themselves. The terms of their reproduction ... are slightly off-beat by good old human standards, in that they involve animal, insect, and inorganic models. In fact they represent a whole array of possible alternative morphologies and 'other' sexual and reproductive systems.

To inform this analysis, there are two examples we wish to discuss, where the implications of digital bodies have been closely linked with medical communities: the Visible Human Project and the Body Worlds exhibition of Gunther von Hagens. Together, these examples encounter the various modes through which the preservation of bodies is enabled via technological process. For the former, it is in the digital architecture of a database. For the latter, it is the immersion of flesh within a physical, preserving nanosubstance. Both examples undertake quite different forms of establishing permanence to biological matter, a defining aspect of the cyborg body. For Body Worlds, the example is enriched by von Hagens' public autopsy, which located the Body Worlds initiative within a series of public spheres where, again, aspects of cyborgism were discussed.

Visible humans in Body Worlds

The digital remastering of flesh for the utilization of medical practice has long-established roots, and technology's capacity to transform assumptions that are made about bodies and how they relate to minds or, indeed, souls is persistent. One only needs to consider the discussions surrounding imaging of the foetus to understand how technology can provoke reactions about the morality of abortion (Campbell 2006). Alternatively, some of the biggest advances in surgery are taking place on the basis of innovation from the computer games industries. These modes of visualization are integral to Haraway's cyborg manifesto and have led Prasad to characterize the processes as 'cyborg visuality' (2005: 292), where digital recording changes the relationship between human beings and machines and allows representational possibilities that are unimaginable without the help of a computer (ibid.: 303). One of the landmarks in digitization was the Visible Human Project (VHP), which was financed by the National Institutes of Health in the United States and undertaken by the National Library of Medicine. The digital rendering of its initial cadaver signified the arrival of a new form of immortality, made possible by digital technology, and, as Kember predicted (1998: 137), it can be seen to have prefigured 'an era of virtual medicine', the exploration of which is the subject of our inquiry.

The VHP drew attention to the major social and ethical issues provoked by representing the body. The project invited questions about ownership over the body, but also how the disorderly body (the initial body belonged to a criminal) could be returned to people as a form of immortalization – a digital taxidermy, perhaps.[11] Moreover, it made visible the relationship between information and matter, and the possibilities that their boundaries might not be very clear at all (Thacker 2001). Dijck (2000: 276) discusses how the VHP brought into focus matters of 'anonymity and representativeness'. The presence of this virtual human 'brought anatomy back into the public domain' (ibid.: 284), and we wish to suggest a connection between this project and the development of digital culture more broadly.

The VHP was conceivable only in the context of digitization, though the themes it raised are comparable to those raised by another recent form of preservation, that undertaken by Gunther von Hagens. This latter example is also a useful case through which the cyborg aesthetic intersects with a range of cultural contexts. Von Hagens' plastinated bodies preserves the body in its natural, recently deceased state. Plastination does not constitute a simulation as such, but is a mechanism for freezing time; not representation, but presentation – almost literally a 'freeze frame', as one would expect from a camera, only the insides of a person are our imagery. Von Hagens' visible bodies occupy a social space that is, in some sense, carnivalesque, reliant on a fascination with the grotesque as a form of entertainment, masquerading as education.

In 2003, the impact of Von Hagens' Body Worlds exhibition in the United Kingdom was reinforced by his notorious public autopsy in London that coincided with the exhibition dates. This event provoked questions about body ownership that engaged a range of interests. Indeed, this range is reflected in the United Kingdom's Channel 4 broadcast of the event, which included commentators from the British Medical Association Ethics Committee, a professor of surgery and an editor of a major current affairs magazine (Miah 2004). At the time, there was a lack of clarity about the legal status of the event and even some uncertainty about the consent process that led to the donor bodies offering themselves for plastination. Nevertheless, the procedure took place, and seemed to have been justified by reason of wanting to make the body visible again and to allay fears about the flesh. Indeed, within the broadcast the medical team made a point of mentioning the value of this public event as a mechanism for informing people about autopsy and, thus, encouraging them to commit to such procedures.

Von Hagens' works and the VHP must be seen in the context of broader processes within media culture, where medicine is engaged. As early as 1975, the summer edition of the *Journal of Communication* reported on the long-standing relationship between 'media' and 'medicine', marking one of the earliest theoretical encounters between the health care professions and media theory. In this volume, McLaughlin (1975: 184) writes about *The Doctor Shows*, in which television doctors positioned themselves as *necessary* outsiders, where they 'can deal objectively with the facts at hand, interpret and shuffle them, and solve all kinds of problems'. In this study, one observes the attempts from those within medicine to adopt the position of expert and authority – to extend their medical gaze – which is similar to the gestures from the medical professions when confronting the Internet. Yet the medical documentary often carries the additional narrative of the spectacle (Dijck 2002), through its implied conflation with body horror movies. In such depictions, representation assumes the various legitimate and illegitimate guises of education and/as entertainment, as a constitutive element of a therapeutic culture (Furedi 2004).

Moreover, recent forms of medical television demonstrate the potential of this media form to corrupt what have been clear, distinctive features of medical television in the past. For instance, the US programme *Extreme Makeover* spawned a series of programmes where health and the game show are combined (Elliott 2003). In this case, cosmetic surgery was undertaken with contestants in a reality television format. A good example from the United Kingdom was the programme *Honey, We're Killing the Kids* (dir. Lock), in which digital morphing is used to age photographs of children who are not eating well. The aged image portrays a bleak future for the children, as the parents look on to see their smiling, happy children photoshopped into malnourished adults with poor life expectancy. Often, this provokes a guilt-laden, shamed response from the parents and the, desired, willingness of them to change their children's eating habits. Yet perhaps the ultimate 'posthuman spectacle' (Waldby 2000a: 24) of medical programming occurs when it transcends all forms of truth making, as one could say of the Dutch production *The Big Donor Show*. Here, the programme began as an entertainment show, not unlike *Extreme Makeover.* In this case, contestants were hoping to win a life-saving organ transplant, and viewers texted in to vote on who should receive the organ. After some days of global news coverage prior to the broadcast, which involved exaggerated condemnations of the initiative (BBC 2007), the programme was aired and, at its conclusion, revealed itself as a hoax aiming to raise awareness about the need for donors (Shaikh 2007). This final case is a useful point of departure for our analysis of the kind of broadcast space occupied by medicalized cyberspace. The examples we use fit within this category of posthuman spectacle, where the medical gaze is now present within a social and cultural sphere in which it is not yet qualified to treat.

3 Cybermedicine and reliability discourse

The emergence of health information and health care systems online has been met with a mixed reception by academics, health agencies, ethicists and the public. Much has been made about the unique capacity for cyberspace to satisfy particular demands for health information (Ziebland *et al.* 2004). Claims about the potential for cyberspace to challenge the relationships between the lay public and public health experts have been tempered by more sceptical discourses presenting a now familiar argument that constructs cyberspace as potentially unreliable and, indeed, a context where misinformation easily gains credibility. Much of what is happening online continues to be framed in terms of its impact on established medical knowledge and the health care professions. In this chapter, we outline the context for some of the discussions we elaborate on throughout this text. We draw upon a range of literature that has begun to highlight the relationships between digital environments and medical expertise to give some overview of the relationship between the medicalization of cyberspace and health expertise.

The reliability discourse about cyberspace reveals how the Internet is framed by a presumption of a knowledge hierarchy. Here, we discuss the notion of the informed patient and health information online (see Kivits 2004) to consider how medicalized cyberspace impacts upon discussions about expertise and health knowledge. In particular, we draw from Nettleton's (2004) work on 'e-scaped' medicine, where she identifies the emergence of a new medical cosmology whereby the sites, spaces and locations of the production of knowledge are changing. In her view, the proliferation of information and communication technologies will influence the means by which knowledge and information are generated and sustained. Throughout this text, we build upon work by Nettleton and others by exploring how knowledge becomes constructed and legitimized within a number of cyberspaces. In particular, we consider the role of cyberspace in the process by which 'health and medical knowledge are being metamorphosed into information and it is circulating beyond the walls of medical schools, hospitals, and laboratories' (Nettleton 2004: 673).

Cyberspace now hosts a variety of new health-related resources. The emergence of virtual health care can be seen in the wider context where health care systems are no longer confined to the doctor's surgery but are, instead, dispersed throughout a number of different contexts (Nettleton and Bunton 1995; Evans *et al.* 2003a). As part of this dispersion, consultations are now increasingly taking place via the Internet (Kedar *et al.* 2003). Responses from health experts to patients' problems can take place privately, for example via email, or more publicly via the posting of advice on websites. These online consultations may provide anonymity, reduce the time doctors spend answering patients' questions in clinical settings (see Spielberg 1998) and decrease the number of visits to clinics (Mandl *et al.* 1998). Moreover, patients may be able to gain expedient advice from specialists more quickly than if they were waiting for appointments with experts in real time.[1] In some cases, online consultations are also tied into partner schemes with health specialists.[2]

Additionally, cyberspace makes possible a vast variety of health material and resources that exist outside of the communicative realm of official health care systems or medical institutions. The expanding range of medicalized resources provides a number of substantive insights into the current cultural negotiations around expertise and health knowledge. As has been stated already, a number of authors are now suggesting that the 'e-scape' (Nettleton 2004) of medical knowledge into contexts such as cyberspace will lead to greater patient empowerment (see Hardey 1999, 2001). Therefore, the emergence of e-health recasts our attention towards the relationships between medical expertise and patients – issues that have been a central focus of medical sociology for some time (see Hardey 1999: 820). This is also because cyberspace is often constructed as a vehicle through which to change for the better the relationships between health expert and patient (Hardey 1999; Gillam and Brooks 2001). Claims have been made that the proliferation of health information and health care online can lead to a more balanced interaction between patient and practitioner in *real time* (Grol 2001; Muir Gray 2002) and greater patient involvement in medical decisions. This drive towards encouraging patient involvement is not peculiar to cyberspace and is reflected, more broadly, in health care policy and practice in certain contexts. For instance, Henwood *et al.* (2003: 590–591) note that in the United Kingdom, health policies such as *Information for Health* (Department of Health 1998) and *Building the Information Core* (Department of Health 2001a) are based on the need for developing 'partnership' relationships between health practitioners and patients (see also Hart *et al.* 2003).

Recent research on the search for online health information indicates how the Internet plays a significant role in establishing that there is merit in the idea of a more informed patient. Indeed, Kivits' (2004) recent qualitative study involving interviews with Internet users provides an excellent critique of the value of the informed patient in relation to searching for health information online. This work illustrates particularly well the limitations of relocating health information online, outside of the traditional medical sphere. Broadly, supporters of the ideals of the informed patient assert that patients may become more empowered during health encounters because of increased knowledge and information. Indeed, ensuring that a patient is informed is a crucial moral and legal requirement of any form of medical care. The benefits assumed in this approach include the patient's more active involvement in their own medical care, as well as the improvement in satisfaction, and in communications between patients and health experts (Bader and Braude 1998; Mandl *et al.* 1998; Spielberg 1998; Czaja *et al.* 2003). It also improves the level of decision making for a patient (Shepperd and Charnock 2000; Czaja *et al.* 2003). Each of these factors is appealing to professionals who continually strive to ensure that they are optimizing the patient's autonomy.

Others suggest that increasing knowledge may lead some patients to challenge the authority of doctors (Hardey 1999; Burrows *et al.* 2000). Evidence suggests that patients may use the information they have gathered from the Internet to guide the questions they ask physicians and health experts (see Ferguson 1997) and that this tells us something about how medicine has changed. As Nettleton (2004: 672) argues,

> [u]nlike the classic sick role relationship where the doctor told the patient what was wrong and what s/he had to do or 'take' to get better, in the information age the patient is just as likely to tell the doctor what might be wrong and outline a range of possible risks, treatments or therapies.

Indeed, the idea that cyberspatial resources would facilitate partnership practice in health is a powerful and prevalent discourse. In what follows, we outline the literature exploring medicine as information, its relationship with discussion on experts and lay public and what this brings to bear upon our thesis on cybermedicalization.

Beyond information

Our position on the possibilities of the informed patient differs from some of the more liberatory accounts outlined above. Our approach to the medicalization of cyberspace is to see its emergence as neither wholly liberatory nor disempowering in relation to health knowledge or patient opportunities. In this section, we outline the literature that has explored the relationship between the retrieval of health information online and the wider impact this may have upon relationships between the lay public and health experts. On the basis of this review, commensurate with the views of Henwood *et al.* (2003: 593), we are cautious about claiming that access to information alone will lead to an empowered health consumer and that this need furthers 'empirical explanation'.

The kinds of socio-medical relations that take place as a result of cybermedicine are inherently more complex than notions of informed or empowered patient would suggest. On this view, various researchers now recognize that we need a much more sophisticated understanding of how Internet users utilize online health information. For example, Nettleton *et al.* (2004: 537) observe that there is a great deal of variability in the 'reflexive engagement' patients have with material accessed within cyberspace. Their position derives from an empirical analysis of e-health use, from which they produced a typology based on the 'informational consequences' of e-health. They suggest that instrumentally reflexive 'expert' patients may be one of many types of e-health users and that they may be using the e-health resources to be 'more discerning in their decisions about: going to see the doctor; making choices about treatments; trying out new treatments; making lifestyle changes; and even self-diagnoses' (ibid.: 545). The potential for that information to be used strategically in negotiations with consultations with health professionals has captured the attention of a number of other writers. However, the relationship between information, knowledge and the health experience implies a more varied set of relations between knowledge and discourse than is implied within current theories of the informed or empowered patient.

While anecdotal evidence suggests that patients are making a more active connection between what they find on the Internet and how they bring that to medical consultation (Eysenback and Diepgen 1999), the potential for patients to use this information to challenge boundaries of health expertise is less clear. In other words, while patients may be gathering endless information online, this does not mean that they use this information to negotiate with experts during medical encounters (Henwood *et al.* 2003; Kivits 2004). Indeed, evidence suggests the limitations of acting out what is referred to as a 'negotiation model' in health encounters (e.g. Massé *et al.* 2001). Further research is needed on the relationship between this health knowledge, patient interactions and the discourses that inform the ethics of such medical encounters (see Komesaroff 1995).

The health encounter has often been described as being dominated by an exchange of biomedical information, with the patient cast in the role of 'a person with disconnected bodily symptoms, wanting a label for what is wrong and a prescription to put it right' (Barry *et al.* 2000). Research suggests that patients themselves may be complicit in establishing this problem, particularly when seeking confirmation from their doctors about information they find online. This is partly influenced by wider discourses that question the reliability and quality of information online. Kivits' (2004: 518) work on the 'informed patient and the case of online health seekers' has begun to provide some useful empirical insights into these issues, suggesting that 'if, at first sight, the trust relationship is destabilized because of failed information provision by doctors, participants do still consider GPs and consultants as their ultimate source of information'. Similarly, Henwood *et al.* (2003: 605) reported 'cases of women who *had* informed themselves regarding their particular health condition and its treatments but when they tried to negotiate with their GPs they had their opinions quite decisively rejected or dismissed'. They also found that some patients felt the need to protect the doctor from the 'informed patient', to avoid exerting extra pressures on an already busy professional (ibid.: 601). The work by these authors indicates that traditional hierarchies may even be reified in encounters between what are seen as more informed patients and health practitioners, when health professionals are positioned as the definitive source to confirm that information. Rather than challenging biomedicine, 'this may lead to a process of displacing and replacing trust in "expertise" and which is accentuated through the increase array of resources available in cyberspace' (Kivits 2004: 519). This position 'implies a belief in hierarchy; somewhere, out at the frontiers of science and engineering' where, in the context of specific kinds of medical problem, there is a conviction from patients that 'a solution must exist' (White 1995: 21). Thus, these stories of medical encounters continue to suggest a tendency to rely on those with 'superior technical skills' (ibid.: 21), as the ultimate source of information.

This developing literature (Kivits 2004; Henwood *et al.* 2003) indicates that cyberspace might not give rise to the deeper transformations of medical encounters that some have claimed it will . Certainly there is evidence to suggest that the rapid growth in health information online has led some patients to become more sceptical about medical authorities. However, the potential to utilize that knowledge in negotiations around medical decision-making processes is, in Komesaroff's (1995: 79) words, framed by 'discursive regularities' and 'constant features of the clinical encounter which distinguish it from all other interactions'. Building on this point, Komesaroff (1995) argues that the negotiations within the decision-making process and the health experts' openness to the contributions, suggestions or experiences of patients are matters of 'micro ethics'. Thus, in considering the relationship between cyberspace, health information and current changes to expert–lay relations, one must remain cognizant of the distinction between 'informing oneself about one's specific health conditions or treatments and being prepared, or able, to disclose what one has found to health professionals' (Henwood *et al.* 2003: 602). Ziebland *et al.* (2004: 3) argue that much of the information provided in cyberspace may therefore only be used in a *covert* manner, so as to avoid risking any 'unnecessary conflict'. Henwood *et al.* (2003: 591) argue that '"information for choice" might better be replaced with the more honest 'information for compliance'''. The role of medical knowledge in this process is captured by Monks' (2000: 31) observation that

> [t]he problem for *patients* is that the very form of medical knowledge, its absolute truth and legitimate statement, renders them simply as an unreliable observer of their own body, subservient to the doctor. Their creative contributions to the diagnosis are made invisible by the very practices through which they and the doctor seek to understand their problems.

The literature alluding to the complexity of an individual's experience with these processes better highlights the relationship between cyberspace, wider medical institutions and constructs of expertise. As Lupton suggests, in their interactions with 'doctors and other health care workers, lay people may pursue both the ideal type "consumerist" and the "passive patient" subject position simultaneously or variously, depending on the context' (1997: 373). This work advances the view that cyberspace may enhance the capacity for one to take up a position of consumerist or passive patient, but one should not read these as static identities brought about through a medicalization of cyberspace. This point is demonstrated empirically in Nettleton *et al.*'s (2004) typology and categorization of different health e-types, which, rather than constructing a typology of individuals, defines the varying patters of *use*. Nettleton *et al.* note that users may, in actual fact, shift from one type of use to another, shifts affected not only by their approach to information gathering, but also by their individual health needs. Significantly, Nettleton *et al.* (2004: 537) suggest that while users might not be instrumentally reflexive, or be able to use this information to negotiate the power relationships between themselves and the health profession, there might be other forms of reflexive engagement with health material in cyberspace. They go on to suggest that 'affective reflexivity' might not involve observable social action, but encompass consequences at an emotional level from feeling reassured, supported or understood. Thus, the 'mundane realities' (Nettleton *et al.* 2004: 547) of e-health use might not offer the sort of challenges to patient–expert power relationships that have been previously anticipated.

Other work highlights how the concept of the informed patient may be problematic when discussing the impact of greater access to information, because of the burdens and imperatives it may place on individuals. The informed patient is considered to be one who *wants* to take action to seek out information for their health. As Green *et al.* (2002: 280) observe, this raises questions about 'who is responsible for the informing and how much information is "enough"?' Such questions connect with broader discussions about how information, risk and choice are being framed within the context of cyberspace. In Chapter 4, we develop these discussions in considering how the search for information connected with the prevention of obesity becomes a moral duty (Lupton 1999b). It reasserts the imperative of health as if it were 'at once the duty of each and the objective of all' (Foucault 1984), imparting a social and moral responsibility to lead a healthy life. As Spoel (2006) argues, this discourse of informed choice is situated within a broader framework of consumerism in contemporary western health care. Within this discourse, patients are positioned as 'consumers' and assigned the burden of taking on an active role to educate themselves about health.

The medical control of health information

Other literature outlines how the impact of cyberspace upon the production of health knowledge and information has been subject to various kinds of moral and ethical debate about the legitimacy of control. In this section, we explore how cyberspace has been subjected to speculative claims that have resulted in a 'reliability discourse' around its function as a source of medical information. Organizations such as the Federal Trade Commission (FTC) and the US science panel on interactive health communication (Gustafson *et al.* 1999a) have warned that much of the information available online may be misleading and potentially harmful. This view is reiterated across a volume of medical literature addressing the potential of the Internet to challenge the authority of the medical profession (Biermann *et al.* 1999). A number of studies examining the quality of websites (Impicciatore *et al.* 1997; Gagliardi and Jadad 2002) and newsgroups (Culver *et al.* 1997) continue to claim that the advice and information available online are extremely variable in terms of quality, reliability and completeness. For example, Impicciatore *et al.* (1997) examined forty websites providing advice on the management of a feverish child and claimed that 'only four adhered to published guidelines'. Within this reliability discourse, Web users continue to be warned about the 'incomplete, misleading, and inaccurate' (Silberg *et al.* 1997: 1244) medical information available on the Web. Such is the extent of this reliability discourse that Coiera (1996) describes the situation as a spread of poor information to the public via the Internet.

In response, attempts have been made to validate medical information, with various organizations claiming to provide ways of assessing and evaluating health information on the Internet (Hardey 2001; Berland *et al.* 2001; Foubister 2000). Wilson (2002: 598) suggests that assessment tools can be 'classified into five broad categories: codes of conduct, quality labels, user guides, filters, and third party certification'. These include the use of gold marks, red flag schemes and seals of approval (Burkell 2004) that help Web users make judgements about the quality of medical information. Rating systems created by both academic and commercial expertise have also been developed, generating criteria by which to assess the quality of websites providing health information. Typically, these rating systems have employed logos related to awards for websites, or seals of approval, which would then be attached to what are deemed to be quality health websites.

It is necessary to acknowledge that there are a number of problems with these rating systems, both with the measurement instruments themselves and with the discourse related to the assessment of health resources in cyberspace. For instance, many of the ratings systems employ 'incompletely developed instruments' (Jadad and Gagliardi 1998) that continue to appear on websites. Researchers and organizations are continuing to explore alternative mechanisms to assist people in filtering out quality health information online, but, as Gagliardi and Jadad (2002) argue, 'whether they are needed or sustainable, and whether they make a difference remain to be shown'. Indeed, despite an awareness of the potential impact that the Internet may have on health care, Ziebland *et al.* (2004: 6) argue that there has been little empirical research that explores 'how people with a serious illness actually use information from the Internet'. However, we would agree with Wilson (2002: 600) that the harder challenge is 'not to develop yet more rating tools, but to encourage consumers to seek out information critically, and to encourage them to see time invested in critical searching as beneficial'.

According to Seale (2005), this preoccupation with the assessment of accuracy, quality, and reliability is structured within a medically defined framework. Discussions on this matter have centred on the authorization of medical expertise.[3] Warnings about misinformation tend to follow the pattern of response by the medical profession found 'in other threatened democratizations of medical information (for example the presentation of medical information on television (Turow 1989))' (Seale 2005: 518). Attempts to control and regulate health information on the Internet have, therefore, been seen as another form of guarantor for 'medical autonomy' as a 'protector of the public interest' (Hardey 1999: 829). Such arguments are based on a belief that the medical community has exclusive access to expert knowledge (Hardey 1999).[4]

Thus far, efforts towards establishing ethical principles to guide assessments of material in cyberspace have been framed by biomedical discourse. This position is implied by Nettleton (2004: 673), who suggests that the response from the medical community to the flow of information beyond traditional boundaries 'reflects its legacy and history of autonomy, paternalism, and altruism'.

These new patient–physician interactions outlined at the outset of this chapter have also raised a number of complex ethical debates relating to online professional practice, informed consent, privacy and equity issues. For instance, Dyer (2001: 7) notes that 'concern about the liabilities of practicing online has been a driving force in endeavours to clearly define the online physician–patient relationship'. Much of this debate has relied upon the extent to which the ethical principles of clinical consultations should be applied to cyberspatial interactions, as Dyer (ibid.) outlines:

> Does a patient have to be seen, examined or spoken to, to have a relationship with their physician? Does a physician consultant to a Web site have an ethical obligation to visitors? Is it dependent on the type of services or contact offered to users at a Web site or the consultant's position with the Web site? What are the boundaries for an online therapist? Can traditional therapy be translated to the Internet, or is it primarily a new form – e-therapy? At what point is there a patient–provider relationship?

As one can see from the above questions, one of the challenges of understanding the value of cybermedicine is in establishing whether it is possible to maintain a robust ethical framework that can govern the actions of professionals who have legal obligations. Should any such ethical framework derive from the ethics (or ethos) of online communities or from principles of medical ethics?

Such deliberations are made more complex in cyberspace because of the ontology of the body, which some consider to be a kind of absent presence. Cyberspace is an environment impoverished of flesh, and yet the emergence of phenomena such as cyberspace results in a continual engagement with body matters. As relationships around health develop in these spaces, one is drawn into body-related discussions, ethics, decisions and reflections. At the same time, the body no longer has to have a 'physical presence', and, as Nettleton (2004: 670) points out, 'the "art of medicine" – embodied within the sight, touch, smell and ear of the clinician with the help of the laboratory scientist – has lost its authority'. Organizations that have contributed to the discourse on these matters draw upon wider notions of medical ethics and attempt to apply these to the context of the Internet. Perhaps most notably, in 2000 an international e-health code of ethics was introduced by the eHealth Ethics Initiative, which is part of the non-profit Internet Health Coalition.

There are proper ethical reasons to deliberate on the potential harm that might be caused through the use of particular health products or services – not least because it is difficult to monitor what is published on the Internet, or to establish robust mechanisms for accountability over what is published (*see* Culver *et al.* 1997). The possibility for misinformation to gain credibility is demonstrated by the Ron's Angels Web-based company (www.ronsangels.com), which purported to sell female ova and male sperm, though it seems to have turned into a promotional tool for Ron Harris' pornographic movie industry. We shall examine this case in further detail in Chapter 6. The difficulty of regulating such sites has the potential to translate into a greater lack of understanding about health and medicine, rather than offering a greater opportunity to inform people (Burgermeister 2004). Moreover, the promotion of medical and health care products and services via e-commerce presents new challenges that can frustrate the objectives of medical service providers. Companies may place increasing moral imperatives upon the health consumer in an effort to persuade people to purchase their products or services. Dyer (2001: 5) found that in many cases 'medical leaders, professional organizations, and medical institutions proved to be less than exemplary ethical role models'. In addition, given the relative freedoms of the Internet, there is evidence of more salient and disturbing features of cyberspatial phenomena such as the selling of prescription medication, and the use of cyberspace as a mechanism for ownership and body trading. Evidence is now emerging of body-part selling that has existed for some years along with in-vitro fertilization (IVF), surrogacy and sperm donation (Miah 2003; Resnik 2001b). Also, the emergence of networks that may be potentially harmful, such as those related to eating disorders, self-harm, cyber-suicide and even cyber-cannibalism give rise to a number of complex ethical concerns that question the democratic 'freedoms' of cyberspace, and ownership of the body. While such cyberspatial phenomena are difficult to define in precise ethical categories, we shall take up some of these discussions via specific cases in subsequent chapters.

4   Virtual governance of health behaviour

In this chapter, we claim that cyberspace has become another media platform through which the governance of health behaviour now takes place. We examine this process by drawing on a number of online resources oriented towards healthy lifestyles that connect with wider concerns about the exponential growth in obesity. Digital environments have been appropriated by various health-promoting agencies and companies as a means of broadcasting health promotion advertisements, tools, services and products. A proliferation of cybertechnologies now enable the lay public to use the Internet to regulate their body size, shape, weight, diet and physical activity. Collectively, these resources can be considered as part of an 'e-health discourse' that combines imperatives associated with 'new public health discourses' with those 'e-society' discourses that are oriented towards consumerism (Henwood 2006). Such resources include Internet sites on health promotion produced by health organizations, intervention programmes, and commercial resources such as health screening, online personal training and weight management sites, all of which play their role in a virtual medical construction of the healthy body. In this sense, we argue that cyberbodies have become inscribed with medicalized information associated with healthism.

Public health promotion in cyberspace

The emergence of healthism in cyberspace has been influenced by online consumerism and a shift in public health promotion from a biomedical model towards a new paradigm of health care based on risk (Nettleton 1996). This trend can be found in primary research in medicine and various health fields. For example, epidemiology asserts that common diseases such as cancer, heart disease and strokes are related to social factors, which, in turn, are related to unhealthly lifestyles. Hence, one may reduce risk factors by engaging in appropriate lifestyle behaviours, such as changing one's diet. This approach to health has been applied to current concerns that western society is in the midst of an obesity epidemic. In the United Kingdom and elsewhere, personal and public lives are increasingly framed and regulated by an incessant outpouring of health messages relating to obesity and measures to be taken to avoid it. The World Health Organization describes obesity as a 'global epidemic', and governments and health agencies have made repeated calls that assert that the prevention of obesity 'should be amongst the highest priorities in public health' (Seidell 2000: 28). There seems little doubt among public health experts, governments and the media that this is a serious problem of epidemic proportions, caused purportedly by inactive lifestyles, fast food culture and changes in our diets, affecting both adult and child populations. This moral panic and its accompanying discourse around cause and effect are now commonly referred to as an 'obesity discourse' (see Gard and Wright 2005).

Although acknowledged as a particularly complex health issue (Bouchard 2000; Flegal 1999; Kassirer and Angell 1998), in the public domain obesity is often reduced to an issue of lifestyle behaviour. Despite the widespread influence of the obesity discourse, researchers across a range of disciplines are challenging some of the claims that have been made about its prevalence, aetiology and effects. Although the facts on obesity are routinely issued with authority and conviction, a number of uncertainties have been found within the primary research on obesity (see Gard and Wright 2001, 2005; Evans *et al.*, 2004; Rich and Evans 2005; Campos 2004). Indeed, Flegal (1999) describes the health consequences of rising obesity levels as at best 'unclear'. The relationship between weight and health is far more tenuous, complex and contradictory than 'obesity' discourse would have us believe (see Evans 2003; Gard and Wright 2001; Flegal 1999). It is worth noting that concerns have been raised over whether the prevalence and seriousness of obesity may have been exaggerated.[1] Others have taken up the task of revealing how obesity discourse can be considered a social construction (Aphramor 2005; Campos 2004; Gard and Wright 2005; Monaghan 2005; Evans *et al.* 2004). In particular, Gard and Wright (2005) argue that obesity discourse brings together uncertain scientific knowledge and is imbued with a complex web of cultural beliefs and ideologies.

Despite these complexities, health organizations, governments and education agencies continue to utilize medico-political technologies to regulate populations through discourses of risk (Gard and Wright 2005; Evans *et al.* 2004; Rich and Evans 2005; Groskopf 2005, Gastaldo 1997). Before we explain how these technologies are being utilized in cyberspace, it is worth expanding on our theoretical use of the concept of *health governance.* In contemporary society, coercive means of manipulating populations using explicit force and oppressive rule of law have given way to more subtle and less certain means of control. Such techniques involve a combination of mass surveillance and self-regulation that Foucault (1979, 1980) called 'disciplinary power'. Individuals and populations are ascribed responsibility for regulating and looking after themselves according to particular criteria associated with what is deemed to result in good health.

As populations have grown and become more fluid and complex, 'an explosion of numerous and diverse techniques for achieving the subjugations of bodies and the control of populations' (Foucault 1978: 140) have emerged. Foucault (1978) refers to this process as bio-power, which serves to bring into view a field comprised of more or less rationalized attempts to intervene upon the vital characteristics of human existence. The vital characteristics of human beings, as living creatures who are born, mature, inhabit a body that can be trained and augmented, and then sicken and die. And the vital characteristics of collectivities or populations composed of such living beings.

(Rabinow and Rose 2006: 196–197)

Thus, attempts to govern people's weight as a solution to the obesity epidemic do not take place through coercion, but via the normalization and medicalization of behaviours. As Groskopf (2005: 41) points out, the World Health Organization's 'global strategy on diet, physical activity, and health' recommends a variety of methods of control to curtail the 'obesity problem', including instruction, surveillance and evaluation. These and other mechanisms of bio-power take an ostensibly educational form via the provision of information and guidelines to equip individuals to avoid 'risky' or 'unhealthy' behaviours (Crossley 2000, 2001). These enable the regulation of populations without actually 'engaging in coercive actions' (Gastaldo 1997: 113). The provision of information around healthy lifestyles draws upon strong moral imperatives that prescribe the correct choices people should make around lifestyle concerning physical activity, body regulation, dietary habits, and sedentary behaviour.

As Ritenbaugh (1982: 352) points out, the terms 'obesity' and 'overweight' have become 'the biomedical gloss for the moral failings of gluttony and sloth' wherein obesity is a visual representation of non-control. Such socio-cultural tendencies are now equally evident in the United Kingdom and elsewhere (Evans *et al.* 2003b; Gard and Wright 2001). In the blame-the-victim culture that such tendencies nurture, fat is interpreted as an outward sign of neglect of one's corporeal self – a condition considered as either shameful, dirty or irresponsibly ill. In effect, this view reproduces and institutionalizes moral beliefs about the body and citizens. The regulation of risk in this way produces both 'population strategies' and 'invidualising focuses' (Bunton 1997: 229). More recently, Halse (2007) suggests that within these contemporary cultures of weightism, one is expected to become the 'virtuous bio-citizen', an expectation that is

based on a humanist ontology of the subject and a deontological ethics whereby personal responsibility for ensuring that one's weight is within the prudential BMI (body mass index) 'norm' is constituted as care for one's self *and* a social and ethical duty to others in society.

Thus, new health discourses associated with the moral imperative to regulate one's weight assert an obligation not only towards oneself but also a social responsibility towards others in a 'moral economy of virtue' (ibid.).

In order to manage the health of a large population in this way, it is necessary for each individual to 'be reached by techniques of power' (Gastaldo 1997: 115), for both the normalization of health and the information on healthy lifestyles to reach across entire populations. To this end, such discourses have benefited from a shift towards what Bernstein (2001a) described as the 'totally pedagogized society', where pedagogical work – which, we add, may instruct us on how to live a healthy life – now pervades every aspect of life, carried out in the media, the home, peer culture and, in more recent years, via a range of new technologies (see also Evans *et al.* 2005; Wright and Harwood forthcoming). In this way, populations are taught about obesity and associated risks via instructional and regulatory pedagogies (Evans *et al.* 2008), which are no longer confined to clinical settings such as the GP's surgery or hospital but are a routine feature of everyday life. A whole range of expertise, across a variety of cultural sites, is being made available under the guise of social support to avoid the risks of modern-day living.

As part of this project, the expanding and ubiquitous presence of networked health information provides a rich context for companies and agencies to promote services related to healthy lifestyles. Many online users surf the Internet precisely to discover such information. According to the Pew Internet and American Life Project Report (2006), of the 113 million Americans searching for health information on the Internet, 44 per cent have searched for information on exercise or fitness, and 49 per cent for information on diet, nutrition, vitamins or nutritional supplements. In recognizing the tendency for the public to use the Internet for these purposes, agencies and organizations have utilized cyberspace as a kind of socio-technology through which to encourage people to engage with healthy behaviours and monitor their lifestyle. There are now a growing number of Internet-based intervention programmes and technologies geared towards changing health behaviours (see Cummins *et al.* 2003: 55) and regulating the body in relation to healthy lifestyles.

The emergence of these cybertechnologies reflects the shift towards a 'multi-sectoral' approach to health promotion (Armstrong *et al.* 2006). Moreover, much speculation continues about its future capacity to provide even further medical care and health promotion. As Cummins *et al.* (2003: 56) observe, in the future, a 'virtual health care system will consist of the *Preventive Web* that will provide information on healthy living and the *Chronic Care Web* that will offer disease management services (COR Health care Resources, 2001)'. Indeed, a number of agencies are already starting to build these virtual systems. For instance, the American Heart Association and the Mayo Clinic are investing considerable resources into developing and marketing Internet-based programmes for health promotion and disease management. In the United States, the National Health Promotion and Disease Prevention agenda 'Healthy People 2010' explicitly notes the potential for Internet programmes to target populations, and has included this as a goal in its agenda (Cummins *et al.* 2003: 54). A specific objective is to increase the proportion of households with access to the Internet, 'recognizing the impact that such media may have as a vehicle for health promotion'. In campaigns such as these, the Internet is targeted precisely because of its ability to reach vast numbers of people, with a capacity to make daily changes to information and statistics.

Cyberspace has become an environment regularly utilized in this 'politicisation of health' (Furedi 2006: 4). In seeking to deal with the impending obesity epidemic, the Internet has been appropriated as the latest medium through which to regulate populations by informing them how they are to monitor both their own and others' bodies through constant introspection and surveillance. The immediacy of computer-mediated communications lends itself particularly well to championing the sort of biocitizen (Halse 2007) associated with obesity, as described above. The Internet differs from other media in that it takes on a more interactive form, partly aided by the advent of Web 2.0 developments. It now provides a vigilant mechanism through which to encourage surveillance of our bodies on a *daily basis*. The Internet is populated with tools that assist with the accomplishment of this project, including counters, tables and health programmes that allow for a more instant and interactive means of monitoring. For example, the 'Get Kids Active' campaign website, www.getkidsactive.com, describes itself as a 'New Zealand based initiative which aims to help provide parents, teachers and caregivers with advice, resources and downloads about getting children physically active in an increasingly inactive world'. One of the key features of this site is the use of a counter to monitor childhood obesity across the globe on a daily basis. Presumably, this is a strategy to validate the need for early childhood intervention around physical activity and diet (Table 4.1).

Providing this information via the Internet enables estimated changes in numbers to be reported on a daily rather than an annual basis. In these digital environments, each individual child's body mass index (BMI)[2] is, therefore, seen to carry more salience since it has the potential to alter the daily figures. The production of BMI tables in this way impacts upon 'the relationship between individuals, populations and geographic spaces' (Halse 2007). The moral obligation on the individual can become much more powerful and can lead to stronger relationship between nations, populations and one's individual weight category. The use of tables comparing the BMI of different nations on a daily basis, therefore, operates to 'deploy a homogenising logic of sameness – a common BMI "norm"' (ibid.).

Table 4.1 Child obesity in New Zealand and the world

	Increase today	*Increase this year*	*Totals to date*
Total child population in New Zealand under 15	43	8,568	948,338
Total obese children in New Zealand	1	135	92,786
Total overweight children in New Zealand	2	510	216,029
Total obese children in the world	1,338	275,387	109,976,230

Obesity counter taken from www.getkidsactive.com

The healthy cybercitizen

Building on the above, such is the moral duty to remain healthy and achieve a suitable BMI that one can observe the construction of what we refer to as the *healthy cybercitizen* who dutifully and routinely observes statistics and searches for information about their health and weight. The healthy cybercitizen is thus expected to utilise these new technologies to remain 'fully informed' (Kivits 2004: 524) about current health knowledge. Indeed, bio-power operates on this very basis, since knowledge needs to be 'gathered on each individual body' (Gastaldo 1997: 115) for it to affect populations. As Kivits (2004: 513) suggests, 'being informed about one's own health also invokes the emergence of a "healthy self" ideal, creating the obligation to reach and sustain that ideal (Lupton 1995; Nettleton 1997), thus driving the endless pursuit of information'. The healthy cybercitizen thereby features as part of the wider project in which the contemporary citizen is attributed with responsibility to

> ceaselessly maintain and improve her or his own health by using a whole range of measures. To do this she or he is increasingly expected to take note of and act upon the recommendations of a whole range of 'experts' and 'advisors' located in a range of diffuse institutional and cultural sites.
>
> (Bunton and Burrows 1995: 208)

As Lupton (1995) asserts, being informed has therefore become a public health imperative, as part of an obligation to be a healthy citizen. It is a key feature of the shift from welfarist to neo-liberal politics within health care (see Petersen and Lupton 1996). Relating this back to our case of obesity, the moral narrative underpinning this means that 'Self control of one's own weight might be described as a form of bioethics' (Bury 1991). Halse (2007) expands on this by suggesting that 'personal responsibility for one's weight is constituted as care for one's self *and* for others and therefore as a moral and ethical duty to wider society'. The increasing emphasis on prevention (of disease) and risk continues to expand the realm of health and medicine not only into the lives of those who are sick but, via processes of bio-power, onto and into the lives of entire populations. Indeed, evidence suggests that the majority of users seeking health-related information on the Internet are searching for preventive, lifestyle-oriented information. For example, of the 60 million Americans who have used the Internet to seek health and medical information, over 60 per cent of these are consumers considered to be 'well' (or, at least, categorized as not ill), who are searching the Internet for preventive medicine and wellness information (Pew Internet and American Life Project Report 2006). In other words, online users accessing networked health information are not just ill patients looking for medical advice or health support. For example, Hardey (2001) notes that some of the most popular UK-based websites (e.g. the BBC (British Broadcasting Corporation) and the NHS (National Health Service)) that offer health advice not only contain information about disease categories but also encompass broader lifestyle advice associated with risk factors.

The commercialization of obesity discourse in cyberspace

Kivits (2004: 520) states that the search for relevant information to reduce 'health risk' appears to be 'a general imperative for contemporary individuals in an information environment' and 'finds a sociological echo in the concepts of reflexivity and the reflexive nature of social life' (ibid.: 513). The author provides a compelling argument that explains how the reflexive management of risk and the popular expansion of the Internet are 'dialectically related', with individuals now consciously, carefully and reflexively 'seeking out' risk-related information to manage their bodies. This notion of self-cultivation draws upon liberal humanist ideas around the possibilities for the individual to be in 'control over his or her destiny' (Nettleton 1997: 208), one who has the capacity for 'self-control, responsibility, rationality and enterprise' (ibid.: 214). Therefore, cybercitizens are encouraged to utilize these technologies to actively shape their biographies and bodies via self-regulation. This notion of the capacity for self-control over weight loss, dietary practice and physical activity is reinforced by consumerist health discourses that occupy cyberspace. Many of the associated resources are promoted on the basis of enabling consumers to 'insure against disease and illness' (Nettleton 1997: 213), including conditions such as obesity.

As Evans *et al.* (2003) notes, this 'risk prevention' approach is accompanied by a massive proliferation of interest in maintaining 'the body' in western cultures, supported in an era of 'flexible capitalism', which is endorsed not only by health care, but also by the health and media industries in the United Kingdom. Cyberspace is an environment in which the amalgamation between the commercial e-health sector and health promotion discourses around weight loss and diet are now commonplace. The e-health sector, which focuses on this form of health promotion, has been 'driven primarily by "for-profit" companies that produce sites for consumer health information and sales of health products' (Neuhauser and Kreps 2003: 16). The growth of these health-related goods and services, Bunton (1997: 235) argues, is influenced by a market logic, which produces both new products and health-conscious consumers. As Pitts (2004: 36) observes, health continues to be a big business in cyberspace, with 'companies like AOL, Yahoo and CompuServe' running 'popular women's health sites that are saturated with advertising'. More intrusive forms of health promotion and commercialization take place via email spamming that advertises health-related products.

The alignment of health with market rationalism within and through cyberspace provides a context for biopower to function in a particularly pervasive form. There are a growing number of commercially based Internet sites trading on the discourse that one can take control of one's life by investing in the body to insure against disease and ill health. These sites offer a range of services and products to enhance a healthy lifestyle, including personal training (e.g. www.workoutsforyou.com) or weight loss programmes (e.g. www.weightwatchers.com, www.fitday.com). For example, FitDay (www.fitday.com) is an online diet and weight loss journal that provides an account to 'enter your daily foods and exercise. FitDay analyzes all your information and shows you daily calorie counts, carbs, fat and protein, weight loss goals, ... long term diet analysis and much more'. Personal fitness training services are also provided in virtual settings where users complete health profiles and health history questionnaires and various assessments online, after which a personal training instructor customizes a programme for the client. In these virtual environments, the client is often then responsible for completing the training and reporting back to the trainer online. Reporting on adherence in this way encourages users to cultivate subjectivities based on the agentic[3] healthy citizen, who not only seeks out health information but also puts that information into practice in terms of actual health behaviours.

In these contexts, commercial companies mobilize their 'biopower' (Rabinow and Rose 2006) by summoning the authority and validity of scientific language and accompanying expertise. For example, the website Changing Shape claims to offer 'online fitness programs that are *verified by research,* which guarantees success among all dedicated clients' (www.changingshape.com; our emphasis). Drawing on scientific knowledge enables health professionals to be seen as more entitled or 'legitimised' to 'examine and prescribe "healthy" lifestyles' (Gastaldo 1997: 116). Another website, called HealthPricer, draws upon a similar discourse of trust and expertise:

> At HealthPricer you can browse for, or search for specific products and we'll provide you with a list of pre-screened trusted merchants that offer that product by price, quantity, merchant rating and other product attribute ... We understand that shopping for healthcare products online is tricky. Not only do you have very specific search requirements, but you also have to worry about online scammers. HealthPricer helps to eliminate all those concerns:
> Trust: to trust us means you depend on us to trust our merchants. We go to great lengths to evaluate and build relationships with our merchants. HealthPricer only represents legitimate merchants.
>
> (http://www.healthpricer.com/aboutus)

Therefore, the Internet represents a crucial context where connections between health and lifestyle become a 'political achievement supported by an institutionalized consumerism' (O'Brien 1995: 193).

Digital self-governance

Many websites like those outlined in this chapter now provide online tools that encourage people to monitor and regulate their bodies in relation to an ever-increasing range of lifestyle factors. Users can undertake health screening, for example via the use of BMI charts and calorie calculators, or target heart rate and smoking cost calculators. Websites associated with physical activity behaviours, for example, typically provide BMI and exercise-level counters as methods of assessment (see Evers *et al.* 2003: 66). These online BMI calculators allow users to enter their height and weight details, which will then generate a numerical weight category. Such information can indicate whether, for instance, one is to be considered overweight or obese. It is provided not just by commercial companies, but also by health promotion agencies and other institutions. For example, InteliHealth (http://www.intelihealth.com), hosted by Harvard Medical School, provides consumer health information on risk assessments, calculators, and online advisers and guides. Similarly, the Mayo Clinic (http://www.mayoclinic.com) has a 'healthy lifestyle planner' providing a range of 'calculator tools' including BMI calculators for kids, and self-assessment tools including a personal health scorecard. Online health screening is also being utilized by various organizations as a way of assessing employees or students. For example, at Stanford University in California a personal health-screening questionnaire is completed online 'by prospective student athletes, to help physicians screen for the risk of sudden cardiac death and other health threats'.[4]

In these contexts, health risks are presented in a calculable form, which has the effect of constructing the body as knowable and measurable by health and medical experts and the general public. These tools encourage people to monitor and survey their own bodies and are productive in bringing about 'practices of self-governance and the governance of populations' (Nettleton 1997: 219). In these processes, physical activity, alcohol consumption, diet, weight, size and shape become subject to surveillance and disciplinary power (Foucault 1988) as individuals monitor and regulate what they consume and how much exercise they undertake. Virtual spaces provide a unique capacity for this form of governance, because of their capacity to reach large numbers of people owing to their interactive nature. They can also act in a more intrusive way than other media, via the growth in spam, allowing companies to send out unsolicited bulk messages to advertise health products and services via emails, messaging services and other Internet technologies. This persistent promotion contributes to what many authors refer to as the 'normalization' of health discourses (Rich and Evans 2005, Rich *et al.* 2006; Evans *et al.* 2004; Evans *et al.* 2003b; Crawford 1980) associated with self-regulation and self-monitoring.

Virtual morality

The practices referred to in the previous section have a number of constitutive effects upon the appropriation of the body and give rise to a number of ethical and epistemological tensions. The emergence of healthism in cyberspace reflects a politicization, commercialization and marketization of health online. The promotion of these resources reflects the occupation of cyberspace by consumerist discourses associated with New Right ideology that assert particular visions of personal agency associated with responsibility and rationality (Nettleton 1997: 213–214). In Chapter 2, we outlined how discourses of the informed patient rely precisely on these concepts of the self. Henwood *et al.* (2003: 597) observe that the assumption underlying the informed patient is that they are someone who '*wants* to take this sort of responsibility for their health, and searches for information in contexts other than traditional medical visits to health professionals (e.g. doctors)'. This constellation of online tools reify the imperative of health, as if it were 'at once the duty of each and the objective of all' (Foucault 1984), to lead a healthy life.

The burden of responsibility is ultimately seen to lie with the individual, to the extent that subjectivity becomes 'culpable' (Fox 1999: 22). One of the problems with this is that, as individuals become positioned as 'consumers' who are deemed responsible for their own body and health, attention can be directed away from wider social constraints of health and illness. Within a medicalized cyber-space, the use of ideals of informed choice is intended to support and promote 'non-authoritarian ... ethics of health' (Spoel 2006: 197). As Hendersen and Petersen (2002: 3) suggest, in this somewhat neo-liberal model of health, con-sumers are expected to be independent, active and informed rational decision makers. Consumerism and the provision of information are presented as a means towards 'personal empowerment' or 'freedom of choice'. This phenomenon can be observed by examining the online diet and fitness industry, or some online health agencies, which draw upon these ideals of empowering people to exercise 'freedom of choice' (Spoel 2006: 204). For example, FitWatch.com is an online service that describes itself as a fitness tracker, and markets itself via the ideals of 'get the data, get the knowledge, get fit'. Its marketing material draws upon a lan-guage heavily inflected by liberal individualism:

> Imagine that you had the opportunity to use a tool which you only needed to use a few minutes a day, yet it would *give you the power and knowledge to help you lose weight and get fit,* would you use it or would you just walk on by and ignore the chance to take control of your life? [our emphasis]

The rhetoric of empowering and enabling 'effectively constructs the individual subject as a "health consumer" in accordance with the model of consumer capi-talism' (Grace 1991: 329). Despite the apparent progressiveness of 'empowerment', informed choice emerges here as 'part of the larger neo-liberal, consumerist discourse and ideology of health care within which this principle typ-ically operates' (Spoel 2006: 198). These tensions are particularly strong in the context of online networked health services and information, where various, com-peting health discourses intersect. While cyberspace provides the public with a vast amount of information and knowledge about health, it is difficult to deny the increasing presence of health resources and commercial services oriented around the health and fitness industry. In this new cybermedical order, 'that which parades as choice is often a narrowing of choice' (White 1995: 36):

> A consumerist ethics demystifies the social determinants of choice by focus-ing on the ideal of individual 'freedom' of choice; it privileges the unidirectional transmission of (ostensibly) value-neutral biomedical infor-mation above other ways of knowing and communicating (Spoel 2006: 197).

Information gathering 'continues the system of biopower' (Groskopf 2005: 42), which augments the messages around 'healthy lifestyles' that already pervade various institutions (popular media, schools, doctors' surgeries, the fitness industry, etc.). While individuals are not forced to act or behave in certain ways, through a blend of disciplinary measures and control techniques, which constitute bio-power (Foucault 1990), populations are being 'facilitated' to understand 'what is good for them' (see Burrows and Wright 2006). Failure to conform to health advice or self-governance does not result in official or legal sanctions; health is not enforced or achieved through totalizing didactive forms of power. Instead, governmentality is achieved via bio-power invoking a powerful discourse of morality, which may induce feelings of shame, guilt and anxiety (see Lupton 1995; Rich and Evans 2005). This form of neo-liberalism calls upon 'the individual to enter into the process of self-examination, self-care and self-improvement' (Petersen 1996: 48–49). Medicalized cyberspace is an environment where discourses of health promotion concerned with lifestyle, commercialization and 'informational medicine' (Nettleton 2004) come together in ways that can enhance these forms of healthism.

5 Cyberpatients, illness narratives and medicalization

Health information in cyberspace is not only produced by medical authorities or commercial organizations; it is also reconstructed through arenas of lay discourse. In this chapter, we explore how Internet users have 'become significant providers of health information and advice' (Hardey 2001: 388) and how medicalized cyberspace is variously negotiated in this process. As Hardey (2001) observes, the Internet is much more open than traditional media and provides a less regulated space for the production of material. Increasingly, online users are creating websites, email groups, electronic networks, online support groups, and so on (Jadad 1999) to share experiences of health and illness. The collation of this material is part of a wider process of 'informational medicine' whereby patients can become *producers* of health knowledge (Nettleton 2004).

Much has already been written about the potential of cyberspace to enable the sharing of illness narratives and for this to act as a form of self-help (Ferguson 1997), or 'computer-mediated social support' (CMSS) (Burrows *et al.* 2000: 106), particularly in relation to terminal illness. Much less has been written about the relationship between processes of cybermedicalization and online patient use of the Internet in relation to conditions that are new or stigmatized ,or where individuals may experience profound illness symptoms and yet have no clinical diagnosis (Nettleton *et al.* 2004). These are particularly rich cases through which to examine the complexities of medicalization, because those who experience such conditions have tended to rally for medical recognition, yet at the same time have tried to make public their very personal, embodied narratives of ill health. Cyberspace has been a significant feature in the formation of networks related to these conditions. We outline how cybermedicalization mediates this process by examining the case of online communities developed by women experiencing persistent sexual arousal syndrome.

Online health communities

It is well documented that people with common problems often use the Internet to enable the formation of virtual communities. Drawing on a range of studies of computer-mediated support groups, Wright and Bell (2003) indicate that many of these support groups might be linked to 'weak tie' network theory.

Drawing on Granovetter (1973), they remind us that 'weak tie' relationships typically take place between individuals who communicate on a daily basis, but are not necessarily close. There are a number of resources included in these cyber-communities, including websites, blogs, email groups/and lists, discussion forums, newsgroups and chat rooms. To this end, the Internet has been utilized as a self-help resource for both sufferers and carers of the ill (Burrows *et al.* 2000; Orgad 2004; Ferguson 1997). Through the ease of accessing patients through digital networks, one can share experiences of ill health in a range of new ways. Many users of these networks believe that their own experiences of ill health are important sources of information that should, therefore, be shared with other sufferers (Pitts 2004: 46). Digital networks have become increasingly pervasive with the advent of Web 2.0, and online support groups and networks have become 'highly attractive to seekers of health advice' (Walstrom 2000: 761). For example, Ziebland *et al.* (2004), in their research on cancer patients' use of the Internet, found that users may garner a great deal of information and find forms of support that might not otherwise be available to them through conventional health care. Yet these spaces are also increasingly being used to find support of a more *emotional* or *personal* nature (see Turner *et al.* 2001) via the sharing of intimate everyday experiences of illness. Online Peer Support for Cancer Survivors, Families and Friends (OncoChat), for example, was developed to offer precisely this form of support:

> Welcome to our home on the Web! OncoChat is a real-time global support community for people whose lives have been touched by cancer. We don't offer medical advice or professional counseling. We do offer lots of hugs and understanding from people who share similar experiences and emotions.
>
> (http://www.oncochat.org/)

Similarly, DIPEx (www.dipex.org) is a charity patient website that hosts a database of 'personal experiences of illness', where visitors can watch, listen to or read the stories (based on interviews) of individuals experiencing particular forms of ill health. The owners of the site developed this resource in response to the growing need for patients to have access not only to medical advice, but also to embodied, experiential information.

Burrows *et al.* (2000) argue that, collectively, these resources might be considered a global health advice network or virtual community of care. These digital environments have been praised for the 'extensive range of knowledge and depth of caring participants may receive from others facing similar concerns' (Walstrom 2000: 762). Similarly, Wright and Bell (2003: 44) suggest that while real-time face-to-face support groups may provide a context within which people can find others facing similar health issues, 'they rarely have the same specificity or singleness of purpose as online support groups when it comes to discussing a particular health topic'. Online communities are particularly useful for those experiencing rare conditions where patients may be geographically distant from one another, or socially isolated, making real-time support groups difficult to form. In this way, cyberspace can transcend geographical and temporal constraints (Wright and Bell 2003) that may impact on how people manage and experience ill health. Elsewhere, studies continue to highlight the other positive effects of these contexts in offering social support, reducing loneliness (Fogel *et al.* 2002; Pitts 2004), improving psychological well-being (Rodgers and Chen 2005) and providing useful alternatives to face-to-face therapy or support groups (Walstrom 2000).

The role of these virtual communities may also be particularly important in assisting people who have health conditions that are rare, or of a sensitive nature, such as substance abuse problems (Wright 2000), eating disorders (Winzelberg 1997; Walstrom, 2000; Dias, 2003; Treseder 2003), urinary incontinence (see Sandvik 1999), mental health (Powell *et al.* 2003) or persistent sexual arousal syndrome (PSAS). This is because computer-mediated communication offers the possibility to control the level of anonymity experienced, making participation in support groups much easier than face-to-face contact for some individuals. This can help to reduce the embarrassment, shame or 'stigma' associated with particular conditions (Wright 2000). For example, virtual communities associated with mental health have been found to make it 'easier for participants to discuss their problems and setbacks' (Winzelberg 1997: 396).

These spaces can offer additional ways for people to connect and share information of both a practical and a more intimate and personal nature. The capacity to 'promote emotional involvement' (Walstrom 2000: 771) may provide particularly empathetic environments in which to foster connections. A number of studies have highlighted how these relations may develop in online health communities. For example, Macintyre's (2003) research on Internet-based endometriosis support groups found that 'respondents preferred the communication of online health communities to other resources such as books or health professionals since the sharing of personal experience indicative of these forms of health communication could not be found elsewhere'. Similarly, in her research on cancer stories online, Pitts (2004: 47) indicates that values that are generated with breast cancer websites and online networks emphasize 'connectedness and empathy over individual survival'.

Illness narratives

The sharing of these stories of illness via the Internet must be considered in the wider literature on health narratives, which has held a long tradition in the sociology of health (see Bury 2001; Kleinman 1988; Frank 1995; Radley 1999). Within these fields, personal narratives have generally been considered to be the 'means by which the links between body, self and society are articulated' (Bury 2001: 281). Bury (2001) notes that ill health is often considered to be a disruption to one's biography, and 'can often lead to a re-examination of personal, familial and work-related issues ... associated with the onset and unfolding of the condition' (Bury 2001: 271). For many sufferers of chronic illness, disease or ill health, narratives may be used as a strategy to cope with this 'biographical disruption' and 'maintain some sense of worth in the face of intrusive symptoms' (Bury 2001). As Frank (1995) argues, in 'the wounded storyteller' people may find healing as they make sense of their suffering by turning their illness into stories. This is borne out by Yaskowich and Stam (2003: 720), who note the importance of conceptualizing the experience of cancer as requiring 'biographical work' and who 'examine the nature of this work in the context of peer support groups'. They describe the 'process of joining, belonging, and identifying with support groups as an important process within [cancer] patients' ongoing biographical work and encompassing a search for a "separate social space"' (ibid.). Similarly, many women have written autobiographical accounts of their diagnosis and treatment of breast cancer (Broom 2001). Pitts (2004: 52) asserts that the 'technologies of writing and mapping the identity of the body-self, such as those we use on the Internet, help us feel in control'. This is partly because the sharing of one's narrative acts as a 'catalyst for recovery', which can have therapeutic benefits (Walstrom 2000: 766).

However, while there are clear benefits to telling one's story, the ability to construct particular health narratives is subject to a process of cultural politics around health and the body. This politicization impacts significantly upon what stories come to be told in particular contexts. For example, illness narratives in western societies are often mediated by the moral imperative to be 'successfully ill' (Frank 1997: 136) and to 'rise to the occasion' when sick. Indeed, Frank (1995) argues that health narratives in western society are heavily influenced by a 'restitution narrative', where one anticipates getting well again and gives prominence to the technology of cure. Broom (2001) asserts that the restitution narrative can be particularly dangerous to women's health, pressing them to construct 'obligatory success stories' (Broom 2001: 250, cited in Pitts, 2004: 37). As Pitts (2004) notes, the expectations towards a restitution narrative may lead to the silencing of other narratives associated with pain, negative feelings and changes in the body (see also Rich 2006). The significance of this is that many alternative stories of ill health may not be made public because of these moral imperatives and the 'fears and prejudices surrounding cultural conceptions of a health issue' (Wright and Bell 2003: 42).

For example, Pitts (2004: 37) suggests that '[s]ociocultural fears and expectations about femininity, women's sexuality and illness encourage a sense of shame and discrediting about breast cancer, [and] can work to "isolate and silence" (Broom 2001: 250) women about its horrible realities'. Digital environments have provided alternative spaces in which women can construct stories that are not based on a 'restitution narrative', but which focus instead on the disordered, painful and repressed feelings and experiences of illness. The incorporation of the social and emotional in these stories may be particularly important for those illnesses that carry specific cultural meanings, for example losing a breast through cancer (Pitts 2004) or living with endometriosis (Macintyre 2003), in terms not just of physical pain, but also of the cultural meanings of womanhood attached to these experiences. The array of women's voices and stories online reveal the power of what Haraway (1991: 175) refers to as 'feminist cyborg stories'. Many of these websites contain a mix of written text along with visual imagery as they document changes in and to their bodies. Importantly, the underlying ideologies embodied by cyberspatial conduits reflect the mediatory nature of cyberspace as it challenges and reframes biomedical constructions of health that may define the body in deeply gendered ways. For example, Batt (1994: 279, cited in Broom 2001) suggests that if many of the stories of the embodied physical experiences of cancer were to be made public, 'we might as a society, move beyond phobia and fantasy to assess what medical research can realistically do and which problems are beyond its scope'.

Cyberspace provides contexts for intriguing and diverse expressions of ill health through new ways of writing text and representing oneself through video and pictures. In some of these virtual narratives and web pages, expertise is no longer medicalized, but derives from experiential knowledge of living with a particular illness. As Hardey (2002: 37) notes, we see a 'blurring in the distinction between the private world of the self manifest in the home page' as it collapses the boundaries between medical expertise and the experiential knowledge of the patient. This brings to the fore the cultural politics of health where medical knowledge 'has "escaped" into the networks of contemporary infoscapes where it can be accessed, assessed and reappropriated' (Nettleton 2004: 674). More intimate, embodied knowledges of the body are no longer necessarily hidden or marginalized by the institutional domains of medicine. In this sense, the 'ill' body can be relocated in cyberspace, and culturally represented in a variety of ways.

Persistent sexual arousal syndrome and the contradictory culture of cybermedicalization

Much of the literature outlined so far has celebrated the capacity for cyberspace to allow patients to develop support networks and construct alternative knowledges of health that challenge biomedical frameworks of meaning. Yet while the Internet offers a less regulated context for the production of alternative narratives, a complex and contradictory process of cybermedicalization tends to infuse online narratives, particularly those that are oriented towards conditions that are stigmatized or undiagnosed. Earlier chapters outlined how the medicalization of many features of social life has become more apparent over the past few decades. Thus, it is hard to find many human experiences that cannot be categorized through medical language. Despite this, there are conditions where individuals may experience profound illness symptoms and yet have no clinical diagnosis (Nettleton *et al.* 2004). The non-regulated nature of the Internet provides a capacity for users to mobilize knowledge of conditions that might be stigmatized or rare, or where treatment or medical understanding of the condition is limited. These include mental illness, AIDS/HIV, chronic fatigue syndrome, attention deficit disorder, Gulf War syndrome, excessive daytime sleepiness (see Kroll-Smith 2003) and persistent sexual arousal syndrome (PSAS). Many of the dissident or marginal discourses constructed by those experiencing these conditions may be seen to lie outside of medical discourse and can be silenced in mainstream contexts. The Internet has played a significant role in the cultural politics of these conditions, operating as a 'form of media activism, to raise the private troubles of people with health problems as public issues through a revitalisation of the public sphere in contemporary post-industrial societies' (Gillett 2003: 608). However, such mobilization is often infused by a process of cybermedicalization that is neither liberatory nor oppressive.

We develop this argument by drawing on the case of networks and support websites for PSAS, which is both a rare and a stigmatized health condition whereby women may experience a form of persistent genital arousal that is unrelated to sexual desire. It is a condition that is often unreported by those experiencing it and provides an interesting illustration of the complexity and ambiguity of personal health narratives online. Many of the women utilizing the Internet for support around this condition have attempted to challenge the way in which PSAS is often stigmatized. One strategy has been to rally for the medicalization of PSAS, so that it may be seen by medical authorities as a legitimate health condition. The role of lay discourse in vying for recognition in this way makes the processes of medicalization increasingly complex. The particular case we examine is a website and support group established by a woman experiencing PSAS who goes under the pseudonym of Jean Lund (see Lund 2002). Having felt isolated and frustrated by the lack of support and acknowledgement of her condition, she set up her own website to chart her experiences, and subsequently took part in a series of media interviews. This website, along with the online support group linked to it, at the time of writing this text was one of the few online resources available to women with PSAS. On her website, Jean describes PSAS in the following way:

> There has been a lot of focus the past few years on diminished sex drives. The causes have varied from daily stress and fatigue to the side effects of medication. But there is a new phenomenon affecting women that has never been discussed. In fact the majority of the medical field itself has little, if any knowledge of it. It is called Persistent Sexual Arousal Syndrome (PSAS). The symptoms are the complete opposite of FSD [female sexual dysfunction] in that women are complaining of a constant need for an orgasm.
>
> (Lund 2002)

One of the first significant features of her narrative, is her quest to investigate this condition for herself: 'Feeling as though I were a freak of nature I started my own research on the Internet trying to find information that matched what I was going through' (ibid.). Jean takes active steps in challenging the pathologization of her condition and goes in search of information that will connect with her embodied and experiential construction of PSAS. By searching for information and by looking for that which 'matched with her', she is simultaneously the informed and critical health consumer while also attempting to resist her pathologized subjectivity. Much of her narrative centres on the need to make public the forms of inequality she experienced. Jean's online story details how she felt stigmatized by the medical community, impacting both on the social construction of PSAS, and also on the way in which she learned to manage it:

> My symptoms began in mid 1995; almost a year after untreated Thoracic Outlet Syndrome (TOS), a compressed nerve in my neck began. During that year I suffered with a lot of trigger points in the lower back of my head, the neck and the scapula area. I also had high anxiety and panic attacks from the pain. Four months before I had surgery for the TOS I noticed an increase in my sex drive. It wasn't a big increase at first but within two months it suddenly became out of control. As soon as I reached an orgasm, it was only a matter of minutes before I felt ready for another. No matter how many I had, I still felt the same way. Alarmed, I made an appointment to see my gynecologist. He ran the usual battery of blood work, checking hormone levels and testosterone levels and did a paps exam. All the tests were normal. He snickered and told me I was 'every man's dream.' Angry and disappointed in his reaction I never went back.
>
> (ibid.)

Stories like this reveal social inequalities in medical treatment and interactions. These encounters are shaped by cultural discourses of gender, heterosexuality, illness and the body. The explicit sexualizing of the condition as 'every man's dream' not only belittles her condition, but reflects how health problems are sometimes constructed through forms of 'disordered femininity' (Broom 2001: 256).[1] PSAS is constructed in a similar way in the popular press. For example, a recent storyline in the British press on one woman's experiences of PSAS was accompanied by the headlines 'sexy Ellie Allen is a girl who just can't say no – because she's too busy saying yes ... yes ... YES!' (Acton and Spencer 2006: 45). Jean claims she experienced a similar reaction from the media, and utilizes the Internet as a context in which to critique these experiences:

> Media from all over the world were clamoring to get an interview and contacted the Globe wanting to get in touch with me. They wanted interviews on how women suffer from PSAS, what it is, how it affects women's lives etc. Although a few other women (who remained anonymous) were quoted in the Boston Globe report, as far as I know, I was the only woman who did further interviews and certainly the only one who had allowed her identity to be known. Did I do it for my 'fifteen minutes of fame?' Hell no! All you have to do is see some of those sensationalized stories and pictures that took hours out of my life for photo shoots and interviews only to be printed with rather embarrassing headlines screaming '**Woman has 800 Orgasms a Day and feels like a Sexual Freak**' to know that I did it only for the attention that PSAS would get.
>
> (ibid.)

These are significant narratives that reveal the inequalities women may face not only within the medical encounter, but also in other features of their daily lives. For these and other women, cyberspace can serve as a vehicle through which to make public the social outcomes of the medical encounter. For many of the women experiencing PSAS, there is a continued stigmatization attached to this condition because of the perceived association between sexual arousal and sexual desire, and the idea that PSAS may be a psychological problem, or a manifestation of being 'oversexed'. On her website, Jean offers an explict counter narrative to this:

> Over the course of the next six years I saw an internist, four more gynecologists, a neurologist, and a urologist, each suggesting I see a psychologist or psychiatrist. ... [T]his is indeed a true medical problem, not a psychological problem. The only psychological problems we face are the ones caused by the frustration of not being able to make it stop, from the drastic changes it makes in our everyday life and from the ridicule we face if we openly discuss it, specifically with men. Even other women quietly turn on us treating us like we are perverts.
>
> (ibid.)

In the extract above, Jean rejects the idea that PSAS may be an imagined condition, or one that may be purely 'psychological'. Efforts are made to mobilize alternative explanations of PSAS deriving directly from the *experience* of the patient:

> [W]e have not found any help or solution and have a hard time getting doctors to listen to us that it is NOT something we are thinking about but our BODIES need continuous orgasms.
>
> (ibid.)

These are significant experiences that 'publicly relate stories about navigating health care' (Pitts 2004: 44) and Jean actively negotiates the meanings associated with PSAS. However, the representation of 'psychological' issues as less important than physical, organic or, in Jean's words, 'medical' explanations, is the means through which a medicalized discourse is reified and constructs a particular subjectivity. Therefore, the presentation of these narratives in cyberspace is an embodied process, as it is 'contingent upon specific health needs' that can 'profoundly impact upon both the emotional and pragmatic aspects of illness experience' (Nettleton *et al.* 2004: 550). Jean uses cyberspace to construct a narrative to explicitly challenge the invisibility of her condition, and reasserts the need for the legitimization of alternative explanations of PSAS that are grounded in the embodied experience of having PSAS:

> The one thing we do all have in common is that none of us are thinking sexual thoughts. PSAS is not brought on by the mind. It is an actual physical disorder and all of us would rather never have another orgasm as long as we live, than live like this. Several think it is something neurological in the brain, I being one of them.
>
> (ibid.)

This case illustrates what Nettleton and Burrows (2003: 177) identify as a juxtaposing of 'diverse types of discourse', as Jean simultaneously emphasizes the importance of aetiology, of understanding 'causality', and of finding a cure to PSAS:

> All I could think of was that maybe now; maybe finally I will get help. Maybe there is a doctor out there that does know what this sexual arousal is caused from and how to treat it.
>
> (ibid.)

Pitts' (2004: 44) work on women with breast cancer is particularly useful for making sense of some of these accounts. She argues that some individuals may, ironically, reinvoke a medicalized discourse, making efforts to demonstrate 'mastery over medical language' and 'establish their credibility' for them to be able to define their own meanings and understanding of health and illness. Part of this involves the process of

> *arming* themselves with information as they try to negotiate the world of high-tech medicine, in a process which not only helps them understand and choose the best treatments available to them, but also to demand that doctors share the power over their bodies and health care.
>
> (ibid.: 43)

Thus, medical language is paradoxically drawn upon to frame the experience and gain legitimacy, albeit to challenge biomedical constructions of their conditions. As Broom and Woodward (1996: 359) note, in contemporary western society 'many individuals and organizations (including employers and insurers) are unable or unwilling to take a person's own word for the fact that they are "really" ill. Some kind of authority is often required to validate a person's claim to illness'.

Within these accounts of PSAS, one can observe a process of cybermedicalization that is taking place in Jean's construction of the management of PSAS. As Pitts found in her study of breast cancer patients in cyberspace, Jean similarly 'appropriates medical discourse to embody her virtual space, presenting her body through the revelations of a medical lens' (Pitts 2004: 45):

> Well it meant they changed the referral from Dr. Jordon to a 'urologist' within their group!! I was pretty pissed off but have been through this all before. In the past I always gave up out of frustration. This time I decided to play their game ... and it wasn't a fun one. I saw their urologist, armed with my print outs on PSAS and Pudendal nerve. He looked at me and asked why I came to see HIM with THAT. I could have been insulted but instead I threw it back in his face. 'Well because I was FORCED to come see you with THIS, that's WHY! I didn't WANT to come see you, I asked to see Dr. Jordon.' He shook his head and sent me away writing a referral to see Dr. Jordon. A week later along came an approved authorization for me to seek mental health!!!
>
> (Lund 2002)

The case of this particular PSAS Internet resource demonstrates particularly well that illness narratives are neither wholly liberatory nor oppressive. The construction of online narratives of illness is mediated by various commercial, medical and cultural discourses around health and the body. For example, consider how a restitution narrative (Frank 1997) is drawn upon in a manner that is ambiguous, complex and often contradictory within Jean's account of her experience of PSAS. In some instances, her story explicitly deals with being successfully ill (Frank 1997), of putting on a brave face:

> I carried on with my daily routine of holding a full time job, running the support group, and focusing on more media attention.
>
> (ibid.)

At the same time, these websites are infused with accounts that emphasize the anger, frustrations and difficulties of experiencing PSAS:

> Just one more doctor I had to set straight. I am NOT bipolar. I even researched it on the web. I'm not. I have a perfect right to the emotions I have been going through. Frustration with the HMO system, frustration towards all the doctors and the time I spend repeating myself to each new one, and then I have trouble going on in my personal life that is causing suppressed anger, rage in fact, that really relates to very hurt feelings caused [by] family members.
>
> I felt absolutely helpless. My lifestyle has changed dramatically. Where I was once a very sociable person and loved outdoor activities, I have become a recluse. I only go to work because I have to support myself. Working is very difficult because I am constantly distracted by the urges ... I rarely socialize because I am constantly distracted and in discomfort.
>
> (ibid.)

Jean's narrative offers a counter-discourse to the traditional medical discourse, which distinguishes the personal/subjective/patient from the scientific/objective/doctor. She constructs a narrative grounded in a patient's experience, from the point of view of the lived body, expressing what it feels like to experience PSAS. This conflicts with the health professional's approach, based typically on the need for health, disease and illness to be understood theoretically on the basis of signs and symptoms. These stories offer some challenge to the dominance of medical knowledge about these conditions. Conversely, Jean also recognizes the need for her condition to be medicalized in order for her to receive some recognition in the form of support and treatment.

These virtual environments provide a context within which it is possible to rewrite social and cultural meanings of certain health conditions.[2] Such cultural negotiations not only are significant for the individual patient, but, in cases like PSAS, have a wider implication for the cultural construction of 'highly political aspects of the body, gender and illness' (Pitts 2004: 33). In addressing forms of inequality, Jean's story of PSAS and other Internet sites on rare or stigmatized conditions may have an 'activist orientation consistent with prior forms of media activism' (Gillett 2003: 619). Networking with others is an important feature of this form of activism:

> I started one [discussion board] on Yahoo and moved her posted messages to my board. So in addition to putting my face out front in media print, I took on making a safe place for women to converge to discuss their PSAS. ...
>
> In the mean time a woman with PSAS and I began e-mailing back and forth. She is not part of the support group but had already found Dr. Leiblum on her own and had been very busy doing research. Dr. Leiblum pointed her in my direction and it didn't take long for us to have a wonderful emotional connection. ...
>
> She asked and I agreed to join her in her research as we began comparing notes. I started her treatment of using prescription **5 per cent** Lidocaine ointment for a couple of days, then using prescription liquid Atropine on a patch in the genital area for a couple of days and then a combination of using both together for a week documenting each day's results.
>
> (Lund 2002)

This sort of exchange of experiential health knowledge has been documented in online support groups for other conditions. For example, in her research on online endometriosis support groups Macintyre (2003) revealed the significance of online communities to build 'collective knowledge' concerning the management of endometriosis. In particular, she found that having experienced frustrations with the medical profession, women used advice from other members of support groups to 'protect their reproductive health'. Collectively, patient-led Internet resources can therefore bring forth 'the prospect of a renegotiated relationship between medical knowledge and lay experience based on shared learning' (Loader *et al.* 2002: 53). Patient-led Internet resources concerned with conditions such as PSAS can take on an ambivalent and contradictory form, and reveal the complexities of cybermedicalization as experienced by various individuals. On the one hand, they publicize experiences that are intimately connected with the cultural politics of gender, the body and health. Yet, in order to gain legitimacy and recognition for these conditions, increasingly these narratives are medicalized by patients themselves. In the specific case of the PSAS networks, online users experience contradictory subject positions, where there is an emphasis on the experiential aspects of PSAS, alongside the use of demonstrable medical knowledge. The emergence of these ambivalent narratives within cyberspace would appear to reflect Green *et al.*'s (2002: 284) observation that decisions and practices of both lay-women and health professionals reflect a 'complicated mixture of health knowledge and advice and embodied cultural experience'. Therefore, these stories might be considered a reflection of the presence of a 'new medical pluralism' (Cant and Sharma 1999) within cyberspace.

In building on some of the earlier considerations of medicalization work in Chapter 3, one is reminded of the difficulties with making ethical claims about the impact of medicalization on behalf of patients. Indeed, there is some evidence elsewhere that suggests how medicalizing 'a condition can have constructive outcomes, especially for people with chronic and refractory conditions such as chronic fatigue syndrome' (Broom and Woodward 1996: 359). As Conrad and Schneider (1980: 247) observe, 'there are many instances in which people have sought to redefine a condition as an illness in order to reduce the stigma and censure that are attached'. Nevertheless, cyberspace serves as a critical artefact in the renegotiation of cultural meanings associated with these conditions, which have these particularly complex relationships with medicalization. In conclusion to Part I, we draw attention to a series of our main points, which should assist the development of our thesis. First, we have outlined the competing expectations that the Internet will bring about categorical changes for the practice and consumption of medicine and health. The medicalization of cyberspace presents a complex series of narratives that frustrate the attempt to neatly discuss its effect. Second, we have considered how discussions about medicalization themselves have undergone a series of complexities that make it difficult to isolate as a static thesis. Medicalization is characterized as a series of illegitimate and legitimate attempts to shape and fashion health from the perspective of institutions and professions, but it is also a process that is endorsed intentionally or unintentionally by patients and medical tourists.

In Part II, we explore in further detail how the body is inscribed through cyber-medicalization processes and how this process should inform the theoretical approach to cybermedicine, considering a number of bioethical issues it presents. We outline a number of cybermedical moments that offer further detail to our medicalization thesis and what this means for a range of literatures that have developed theoretical work on posthumanism, public engagement with science, cyborg theory, legal studies of cybermedicine and the relationship between ethics and cultural studies. Many of these debates are pertinent to what some authors have described as an emerging biomedicalization (Clarke *et al.* 2003), though we stop short of using this term, since our study is located less in biological modifications and more in considering how the digitization of biology is the context for this imminent future of lifestyle medicine.

Part II
Cybermedical bodies

6   Partial prostitution

The digital culture retrospective in Chapter 2 outlined the various ways in which discussions about the body frame analyses of medicalized cyberspace. There, we indicated that Part II will analyse a number of cases and examples of the issues raised by this process and what it tells us about the developing relationship between medicine and digital culture. Specifically, critical concerns have emerged within Web studies associated with the vulnerability, ownership and commercialization of bodies, each of which responds to central areas of feminist concern. Within cyberspace, the body has become re-owned, bound by the need to perform identity. Our cases in Part II articulate instances where concerns have arisen about such performances. The core concept of consideration throughout Part II is the emergent *posthuman body,* a political positioning of the human condition as perpetually in flux and inextricable from technological systems. Our articulation of a posthuman body should not be seen as an essentialist claim about what it means to be human, since continual change in itself is too abstract a characteristic to be meaningfully descriptive. Moreover, such a position would neglect to take into account the relative permanence of specific periods of the bodily condition for individuals. For instance, if one considers modes of communication as an indication of how humanity has undertaken various changes in language systems but also in the various media that make communication possible, the claim would be that these modes have changed. However, it is also obvious that specific modes of communication have remained the same, despite these changes; email has not replaced the telephone or face-to-face communications in many aspects of life. Moreover, people often spend their entire lives without making the transition from one mode to the other, which is in part why discourses of transformation often invite scepticism.

We draw together these themes by identifying a number of cybermedical phenomena that have become characterized as disturbing or deeply worrying in a range of discourses (governmental, medical and media). In doing so, we reveal how the cyber news story is accompanied by expressions of 'anarchy and chaos' (Sandywell 2006: 47), that shape moral evaluations of online activity. This discourse embodies the characteristics of Kelly's (1994) thesis on the co-evolution of machines and biology, which helpfully reveals the broader context of our claims about cybermedicalization. It consists of a perceived instability and vulnerability arising from the networked society that is reflected in the contemporary human condition, made lucid by *internal* technological change. Thus, Kelly's 'new biology of machines' is also an infestation of biology by machines, the manifestation, for Haraway, of a *new,* 'soft' cyborg.[1] One of the clearest examples of this imminent collapsing of boundaries is the work of Kevin Warwick, whose (disputed) self-authorship as the *first* cyborg suggests a posthuman or post-robotic synergy between the natural human and automata, which boldly claims that 'life is the ultimate technology' (Kelly 1994: 165).[2] These prospects are also prescient in the work of cyber-body artists such as Stelarc (Smith 2005), whose early suspensions remind us of the entrenched historical context of internally invasive transformations. The rupturing of his skin by body hooks neither refers back to ancient rituals of body piercing nor attempts to convey social demarcation. Rather, it occurs as a challenge to the claim that such ruptures in contemporary times must be tied to the development of technology.

The cases discussed in this chapter articulate moments where non-medical Internet entrepreneurs have created new medicalized cyberspaces, which have become a focus for debates about the problems arising from the Internet. As such, they do not constitute attempts from the allied medical professions to consider how the public might use the Internet to communicate issues related to medicine and health. Among these examples, the authoritative expert voice has become jeopardized through social software. In these cases, the anarchic potential of online communities is modest at best, particularly when many of the major platforms are owned by either old media or the older new media (e.g. Google's purchase of YouTube). Even in the context of fictional spaces, governmental processes emerge, as was exemplified by the virtual rape episode that took place within the online text-based game environment LambdaMOO (Dibbell 1993; Mnookin 1996; MacKinnon 1997). In 2007, this case was updated by a similar story within the graphical online game Second Life (Lynn 2007).

In 1999, there were at least three significant moments that reflected the complex ways in which cyberspace was becoming medicalized. The first arose in relation to human cloning. The second was the emergence of pornographic film director Ron Harris and his Ron's Angels enterprise. The final case was the episode of a human kidney auction on eBay. Each of the cases gave rise to terse debates about technological control and provoked a number of strong moral reactions about the value of the Internet as a conduit for information and, indeed, social organization. In different ways, they emphasized the limitations of media discourses surrounding science, medicine and technology and, perhaps, reflected the boundary testing that is so often associated with Internet usage. More specifically, they demonstrated the place of moral debate in contemporary cultural discourses, made explicit by Zylinska (2005) and, in particular, how the body is appropriated through these discourses. Indeed, this is the focus for the chapter.

In sum, this chapter investigates the historical development of the digital body and how its presence has been tied to concepts of ownership, commerce and exploitation. However, the partial prostitution we describe is not meant to have a pejorative connotation. Rather, we discuss it as a necessary function of the body-as-product that emerges through its digitization. Individuals with digital presence are all participants in partial prostitution, on some level. Cyberspatial phenomena have brought into focus the moral implications of commercializing the body, a concern that arose some years ago (arguably, since the 1950s) when various attempts at organizing paid organ donation gave rise to much criticism for the manner in which they were handled.

The eBay auction for a human kidney

The rise of eBay is fast becoming a distant memory, as it has come to occupy a meaningful commercial space for many online users, as either vendors or buyers. Yet it is important to remember that its development performed a crucial function in establishing one particular part of the Web's history, especially as concerns the mode of engagement encountered by the individual user. eBay contributed to the range of possibilities offered by the Web in three important ways. First, it offered a mechanism for the sale and resale of all entities on a global user-to-user level, previously unencountered. Second, it presented a peer review system of evaluating individual users' contribution to the community, by allowing members to rate and comment on their transaction encounters.[3] This became constitutive of individuals' reputations and symbolic of their trustworthiness. It also functioned as a tacit social contract, whereby participants saw the value of feeling obliged to leave comments about transactions. Third, it enabled career opportunities for entrepreneurs, without eBay's functioning as an employer as such. These factors were not unique taken in isolation, but as a combination they were innovative as far as the Web was concerned.

However, these details are only partially relevant to our consideration of eBay, which is more specifically about a particular occurrence within eBay's history: the auction for a human kidney. One of the more controversial concerns about the Internet has been its capacity to facilitate the trafficking of organs, though one might question whether the Internet has any special relationship to this phenomenon, which we know exists elsewhere in various forms. However, the eBay auction of a human kidney raises a number of questions about the role of the Internet, its function as an open space of human sociability and its capacity to act as a regulatory authority. Our analysis allows for this tale's function either as a fictional occurrence – something that was staged by a participant – or as a genuine, though never realized, event. Moreover, it is constitutive of our overall analysis that fictional tales contribute to the folklore of the Internet and the range of technological potentialities that might be written into its design. Indeed, we will encounter various similar examples within this part of the book.

What interests us about the auction is the range of conversations it provokes about changing values associated with health and the proper domain within which these discussions might take place. The eBay auction of a human kidney establishes the terms of this problematic and neatly captures the range of potential regulatory challenges that the Internet presents. One might characterize this instance as the beginning of an array of Web-related organ trafficking services that are likely to emerge.[4] The authenticity of the case, as an instance of illegal organ trafficking, facilitates a particular imagination about the Internet that is not otherwise provoked. In some sense, the instance is an exercise of fiction, which, nevertheless, contributes to the overall expectations people have about technology generally and the Internet in particular.

The details of the eBay auction for a human kidney are unambiguous. In 1999, an unprecedented lot was announced on eBay, which led to a number of debates. The auction was short-lived, failed to conclude, and was quickly removed from the site after it was made known to the company (Boyd 2002). Nevertheless, the specifics of the occurrence are intriguing. As Schafernak (2000: 901) notes, the bidding 'reached $5,750,100' and 'in response to an about.com on-line poll conducted the following week, 69 per cent of respondents thought it should be legal to sell one's own kidney'. The example engenders the pre-millennium anxiety surrounding debates about Y2K. The case was one of the clearer instances of the Internet's lack of control or regulation from the state. However, the connections should be made at a deeper level, between organ trafficking more generally and its spread across the Internet.

A central concept related to organ trafficking concerns 'borders', as is true of wider legal issues surrounding medicine in a global context (which we also consider in Chapter 7). The Internet constitutes a rebordered, non-geographical digital-scape, and it is the struggle over borders that concerns many involved with Web development. For instance, in Chapter 7 we shall take up issues of ownership over domain names, copyright and 'copyleft' (Heffan 1997), debates that are all critically about ownership of some kind: ownership over distinctions between what is public and what is private. Where this debate concerns parts of *real* bodies – *real* organs – the conversation engages a range of governmental organizations and professions. Thus, the eBay auction of a human kidney was one of the early, monumental episodes in the medicalization of cyberspace, which was exemplary in its drawing in a range of medical professions as interested netizens. Its alignment with a criminal underworld reinforces – falsely – the discourse on its status as a disempowered, dubious act, most likely from a position of desperation and vulnerability.

Not another human clone!

In the same year as the eBay human kidney auction – two years after the cloning of Dolly the sheep – the media announced that the first cloning of human cells had taken place and that the first cloned human could soon be born (see BBC 1999). The legal implications of this are quite well known and we will not rehearse those arguments here (Bonnickson 1997; Harris 1998; Human Genetics Advisory Commission 1998). Suffice it to say that there remains widespread resistance to reproductive cloning, particularly where it would involve bringing to term a human baby. Indeed, even reproductive cloning to certain stages of cell division continues to meet fierce resistance from pro-life groups.

While cloning technology relies on a range of digital technological systems, our point is not simply to discuss this reliance. Rather, the example helpfully situates debates about the emerging technological cultures of Internet use with a range of other *fin de siècle* questions about what technology might bring. For instance, in the BBC *Panorama* programme on 'the first human clone', the Raelians were portrayed as being accessible via the Internet, as if the marginality of this group is conveyed by its online status. More importantly, human cloning is one of the paradigmatic cases through which popular imaginations of the posthuman have been conveyed in recent years. However, of particular relevance to us are the inaccuracies of these claims and the irrelevance of truth in the construction of such possibilities.

The case of the first human clone also reveals something about the inadequacy of top-down authority and expertise in new media culture, where, as Nerlich and Clarke (2003: 44) discusses, 'so-called "maverick" scientists can play a distinctive and influential role that is quite different from their orthodox colleagues'. In the case of cloning specifically, Nerlich (ibid.) reveals how such scientists

> claimed to be able to achieve the as yet unachievable, but a type of 'unachievable' that has repeatedly been 'achieved' in science fiction: the cloning of humans. The debate this stimulated with other scientists, the media and the public tapped into well-established cultural representations of cloning and increased fears about the ethical, legal and medical risks associated with human cloning.

Since 1999, claims about the first human clone have been made a further three times, and yet none of them seems meaningful.[5] The world has still not seen the first human clone, and most likely it never will. By this, we do not mean that the cloning of a human will never take place, or, indeed, that it has not already. Rather, the reason why we will never see a real human clone and, in part, the reason for raising this example, concerns the way in which science is imagined or made metaphorical via (new) media. The cloning of humans, as it is described in the lay imagination, will never happen, because the science does not promise any such possibility. Armies of clones – which presumably imply some overtaking of the non-cloned human species – or copies of specific celebrities will not be made via cloning technology. To assume such a prospect is to overstate the role of genes in the development of human characteristics – from simple facial expressions to complex behaviours. To take seriously such possibilities and, indeed, to liken them to what took place in Nazi Germany, as is often done in bioethical rhetoric about such technologies, is to be grossly complicit in technological determinism and, more importantly, misdirects the value of being vigilant towards new health care policies surrounding reproductive freedom.

Nevertheless, the overshadowing spectre of these prospects is important to take into account, as it shapes the discursive frame that emerges around any new technological culture. Indeed, it relates particularly to our third moment of 1999 where science invaded the cultural and moral sphere: the phenomenon of Ron's Angels.

Egg Pharm, Inc.

Ron's Angels was another example of the Internet's capacity to generate its own political and cultural forces. The website gave rise to a wave of media and academic attention as it purported to host auctions for sperm and ova – something explicitly forbidden on eBay (BBC Online 1999). In short, participants could bid for the best genes for their future children, and the highest bidder won. Ron's Angels appealed to the burgeoning biopolitics of human modification, where prospective parents are offered new freedoms to determine the characteristics of their prospective children. The case is interesting, again, for various reasons. First, one cannot disconnect it from the rise of debates about the prospect of creating designer babies, which coincided with the end of the millennium and the race to map the human genome. This decade was an era of new frontiers and bioprospecting over the potential for genetics to enable all kinds of radical opportunities. Moreover, these discussions were fuelled by the ongoing concerns about genetically modified foods, where the science of genetics met the culture of consumption. Second, the appeal of Ron's Angels was in the reduction of these prospects to present-day technology – the combined technology of egg harvesting and sperm donation with the democratized technological space of the Internet. It constituted a decisive individualist act through which the propagation of one's interests – rather than one's biological identity – could be bought. Indeed, the values that it espoused were made explicit within the website:

> Beauty is its own reward. This is the first society to truly comprehend how important beautiful genes are to our evolution. Just watch television and you will see that we are only interested in looking at beautiful people ... our society is obsessed with youth and beauty. As our society grows older, we inevitably look to youth and beauty. The billion dollar cosmetic industry, including cosmetic surgery is proof of our obsession with beauty.
>
> What is the significance of beauty? It has been reported that young babies prefer to look at a symmetrical face, rather than an asymmetrical one. Beautiful people are usually given the job of selling to, and interacting with society. This continues throughout our adulthood. The act of creating better looking, or in some organisms, more disease resistant offspring (known as Genetic Modifications), has been taking place for hundreds of years. All genetic modifications serve to improve the shape, color and traits of the organism. 'Aroma and attractiveness is nature's shorthand for health and hardiness'. If you could increase the chance of reproducing beautiful children, and thus giving them an advantage in society, would you?
>
> Any gift such as beauty, intelligence, or social skills, will help your children in their quest for happiness and success.
>
> (Harris 1999)

The Ron's Angels website provoked responses from government and health care institutions about the legitimacy of new commercialized reproductive technologies, and there was widespread condemnation of this new organization. Months after it emerged, the website boasted that over '5,000 articles' had been written about its emergence, and a range of major media organizations drew attention to it. For example, Resnik demonstrates how this new media event functioned as a catalyst for discussions about the ethics of human egg commerce: 'Perhaps the auction was simply a gimmick, but human egg commerce is a serious and rapidly expanding business' (2001b: 2).

To this degree – and a third reason for our interest – the case of Ron's Angels exemplified the concerns about medicalized cyberspace and the various complexities of this process. It was an indication of how the Web constitutes an anonymous, authoritative space, where good design skills often confer a legitimizing mode of authority and authenticity. The emergence of medicalized cyberspaces upturns established social orders and, in the context of medicine generally and reproductive technology specifically, this is no small matter. This kind of instance gives rise to the pressure to control information and the need for legitimate authenticating interventions from the medical profession in cyberspace as discussed in Chapter 3. Yet it is also such developments that reveal the inadequacy of institutional direction on matters related to culture, such as the role of medicine in society.

When the Ron's Angels website emerged, it had the presence and appearance of, then, professional-looking sites, and it appeared to be a genuine and serious initiative.[6] It is only when considering more closely what it aspires to achieve and by following its development over a period of time that one becomes aware of some questions over its sincerity as a liberatory device for ultra-careful parents. Had Ron's Angels been a more sincere attempt to defend procreative liberty, then one might have found it more interesting, but it is the sub-text to this project that raises questions, both about the substantive matters related to the enterprise and, more importantly here, about how the Web allows such initiatives to flourish. Ron's Angels was one of many sites that – unknowingly, we suspect – subverted established cybersocial structures. What was once a venue for entrepreneurs to make their dotcom millions was now a space where anybody could appear credible, important and enterprising. The bewildering part of the Ron's Angels phenomenon was that it continued to be taken seriously. Even today, its website boasts $39.2 million in sales for the years between 1999 and 2004. Yet it seems now that the attention Ron's Angels received not merely was misplaced – no great statement about procreative liberty was really attempted – but also distracted us from the main enterprise of Ron Harris: pornographic films. This, again, enriches the case for our current analysis, as we will in later chapters emphasize the interconnected questions about sexuality and gender that are present in medicalized cyberspaces. The Ron's Angels website de-genders the donation of genes by, for instance, failing to convey the relative contributions of male and female donors in this new commercial venture. While the prices for each were some indication of this difference, this did not wholly communicate what it was that each must endure.

As the close relationship to Harris' other industries became clear, it also appeared as though the donors were hand-picked from his casting list and thus were not quite the kinds of superhuman that might have been expected by at least some critics. Yet the presence of Ron's Angels responded to and brought into question the legitimacy of the Internet and its capacity to offer new, liberal opportunities. However, important questions need to be asked about the nature of this 'prostitution' and how it is made meaningful through the Internet. Soon after the Ron's Angels development, the United Kingdom's *Sunday Times* newspaper ran a story about a female Oxford university student seeking to auction her ova (Harlow and Gould 1999).

It is intriguing that an initiative like Ron's Angels would have such an impact across a range of medical networks and institutions, though it is necessary to follow its development to understand its significance. For example, one might develop an analysis of how online presence transforms the boundaries of media production by constituting new kinds of fictional spaces that are not beholden to the kinds of journalistic rigour of mainstream press publications.[7] Given the discussions surrounding Ron's Angels, one might wonder both at the way in which an online presence is given authority by a range of media and political actors and at how this contributes to the discussions about the nature of credibility online. Indeed, this is one of our central themes, and it has been of significant concern to a vast amount of medical literature interested in how the Internet is used to provide information to, particularly, vulnerable groups such as patients. Ron's Angels emphasizes the lack of reliability, but also the possibility of challenging dominant ideologies by its existence within a medium of ambiguous realness. In short, because it is not possible to distinguish between different forms of institution online, we have precisely the problem of trust and a 'loss of orientation' (Virilio 1995). While we disagree with Virilio's pessimism over this, it is important to take into account how orientation functions differently within online environments.

These three examples occupy quite different conceptual spaces within our analysis of cyberspace's medicalization compared with the later chapters on communities of eating disorder. The distinctions respond to the earlier questions about the meaning of community, thus informing one of the core discussions within Web studies. The absence of community, or, perhaps, the imagined community of eBay users or of parents seeking donor genes, contrasts with the community-led structures of eating disorders, which we shall explore further in Chapter 8.

The examples of egg pharming, online organ sales and human cloning also provide a context through which one can draw together the distinct areas of cyber-cultural theory and bioethics. As Kitchin (1998: 85) notes:

> Cyborg-rendering technologies have opened a whole can of ethical worms. The body is being transformed into a site for a series of ideological skirmishes (body politics) relating to abortion rights, fetal tissue use, AIDS treatment, assisted suicide, euthanasia, surrogate mothering, genetic engineering, cloning, sex-changes, cosmetic surgery and disability issues.

To be clear, our analysis of medicalized cyberspace traverses these two areas of inquiry within which medical sociology is located as a proposition to their integration. Emphasizing the importance of care over justice, feminist bioethics isolates the contradiction about whether reproductive technologies are liberating women or further enslaving them to their bodies (Mahowold 1994). This question is further problematized by the claim that the abhorrence felt towards body parts is a consequence of a patriarchal discourse on the body (Pence 2000).

Among the many problems raised by egg extraction (taking) and sperm donation (giving), one that has failed to gain much attention is the relative sacrifices men and women would make in providing their donations: the female, placed through an uncomfortable procedure of egg harvesting; the male, seeking an orgasm. Both were announced through the Web and both are instances of fictional histories made possible by new media and the saturation of Web news. The first human cloning was also claimed in 2000, 2001 and 2002, and Ron's Angels is merely one example of body-part sales that have existed for some years through IVF, surrogacy, and sperm donation (Miah 2003; Resnik 2001b). These technologies have captured public attention because cyberspace has the capacity to refashion news and re-invent reality. They demonstrate how pseudo-fictive acts can give rise to real-life consequences, notably the many thousands of articles written about Ron's Angels. Also, by misfortune, the juxtaposition of this liberalizing initiative with a pornographic machine brings into question how one should treat medicalized cyberspace. The result is either a technology that is far in advance of its users' identity boundaries, or a technology distorted by its inherent tendency towards capitalizing on cultures.

To reinforce our earlier point, this example reveals the tendency for the Internet to provoke core feminist concerns about vulnerability, an ethics of care, and the propagating of patriarchal values via technological solutions to alleged problems. In this case, the alleged problem is the challenge one faces as a prospective parent to attempt to optimize the advantages one's child will have in life. Presumably, purchasing the best genes is believed to extend this advantage, as is the promise offered by Ron's Angels. The Internet's contribution to these forms of bio-prospecting is its capacity to offer an authoritative and legitimizing space through which marginal or radical ideas about the regulation of medicine can be made visible. Moreover, it presents a wholly technological and genetic essentialist stance on what might be regarded as the enhancement of humanity, to the exclusion of any role for nurture. Yet an integral part of its value is its having arrived at a time when such claims seemed like sensible options to humanity. Resnik (2001b: 4) notes that we might defend egg commercialization on both radical and liberal feminist bases: 'Liberal feminists argue that egg donation can be justified on the grounds of reproductive freedom, while radical feminists argue that egg donation is patriarchal and exploitative.'

In response, the medicalization of cyberspace is provoking a virtual (re)appropriation of the (female) body. Owning humans commercially and symbolically, the Web entails an identity bind that hitherto has not been addressed by literature in either cyber-feminism or cybercultural studies. Indeed, cyberspatial phenomena have brought into focus the moral implications of commercializing the body. However, the mechanism of ownership and body trading is far broader than it previously has been. Increasingly, the body-as-product is not simply symbolic but less visible. The locus of control resides with the user in an intuitive sense, but can be seen as a product of the cyberspatial interface. Cyberspace has become a critical medium for constructing these ongoing discourses, which rely on provocation and disgust as a means towards generating meaning and authenticity. The formal structures of the Web authenticate actions by constructing ambiguous spaces, where such events as cyber-suicide (Rajagopal 2004) and cyber-cannibalism (Lander 2004) are recent examples of how bodies have become visible spectacles.

7 Biological property rights in cyberspace

In the context of the shift from *identity tourism* (Chapter 2) to *body trafficking* (Chapter 6), there is even greater concern about the inability to control (bodies within) virtual worlds. However, this should not generate a special kind of anxiety. Instead, medicalized cyberspace should be seen as reconstituting traditional questions about control, the individual and the state. Moreover, it is necessary to take into account that these processes of transforming bodies are imbued with moral narratives that imply a dubious obligation of fear. On this matter, we again urge caution over claims that would reinforce the rhetoric of moral panic about these developments. The two sets of claims about partial prostitution – that medicalized cyberspace is inherently a commodification of body parts and products and that it invokes particular kinds of moral expectations that are often founded in imagined media events or non-media events – give rise to discussions about what rights one ought to have in cyberspace. Should people be permitted to trade their bodies, identities or, indeed, their genes online? Are there specific kinds of regulations that ought to ensue within virtual worlds over this kind of practice? Alternatively, are the bioethical implications of such services different from those of non-cyber medicine, warranting a revision to both the legal structures and the ethical frameworks that govern the development of such facilities? In short, can we argue on behalf of a *virtual exceptionalism* to how bioethics is dealt with within cyberspace?

This chapter emphasizes specific cybermedical cases, particularly the regulation of pharmaceuticals online. Our interest also extends from the previous chapter to considering the legitimacy of *reproductive rights* claims in cyberspace, where we use this term to offer a direct link to the previous cases, but also to introduce analogous debates in the context of intellectual property rights. First, we consider how reproductive rights have been debated and structured within and around cyberspace and what similarities there are between intellectual and biological reproduction rights. Second, we explore what legal issues medicalized cyberspaces provoke, before concluding how cyberspace constitutes an end point for how society makes sense of the technologies of medical expertise. Finally, we consider how these issues inform our understanding of the relationship between biology and computing as a form of prosthetic encounter.

Reproductive rights in Cyberspace

The concept of reproduction in online environments encounters a dual problematic. A first understanding – which emphasizes the contextual matter of the human cloning discussion – involves the digital reproduction of texts, images and film. The *cloned effect* that is enabled by digital reproduction, and which distinguishes it from the physical matter of analogue, again responds to our interest in questions of legitimacy and authenticity.[1] An examination of this is offered by Baudrillard's notion of simulacra, though our focus diverts from the possible crisis that this implies over meaning and originality. Rather, our interest is a second kind of problematic, which involves understanding how reproducibility – biological *and* digital – has structured discussions about ownership and entitlement in contemporary society and politics. These concepts – ownership and liberty – are shaped by biological metaphors that are located within a traditional mode of embodied action. However, these categories now have only a partial bearing on how reproduction must be understood in the form of virtual interactions. If the earlier example of Ron's Angels conveys the possibility of (Web-) designed procreation, then this chapter considers discourses – both legal and ethical – on the entitlement to act upon such opportunities.

We analogize the right to reproduce – and, in effect, publish or give life to – images, text and other communicative media in the Internet to the right to undertake the kinds of activities mentioned in the previous chapter. We argue that there is an originary moment that occurs in the creation of both text and life that is also inextricable from the technological means through which each is enabled. These discussions are made more interesting by the rise of Web 2.0 platforms, which further challenge the legitimacy of reproducing digital content.

Intellectual and biological property rights

An analogy between *intellectual* and *biological* property rights has not been discussed much in cultural theory. Indeed, Thacker (2003: 48) notes that 'there has been relatively little exploration of the ways in which an informatic paradigm pervades the biological notion of the body and biological materiality itself'. Yet there are various associations that have been made that are suggestive of its relevance. While our interest – in support of Thacker – is not to further claim that the body has become mere information, we are interested to understand how this claim has some bearing on the language through which rights claims over the body are understood. In short, we extend Thacker's claim about the term 'biomedia', which explores the equivalence between genetic and computer codes, to the cultural and regulatory discourses that surround each. This equivalence extends beyond the 'materials and functions' (Thacker 2003: 52) of biology and computing to a discussion over 'what a body can do' (ibid.: 53) as a legitimate and legitimizing act.

Today, one of the pervading conversations about the networked society involves matters of ownership and intellectual property. As an increasing number of Web-based platforms emerge that compete with established distribution channels of broadcasting and publication, the question arises as to who owns information and what standards of control operate to govern this mechanism of authorship and publishing. Such enquiries encounter discussions about what is public or private online and what the role of the media is when they are no longer required to convey information that would otherwise be inaccessible.

Equally, one of the central conversations about procreative technologies involves questions of ownership over biological matter. More specifically, emerging biotechnologies encounter questions about whether individuals have the authority to alter themselves or, indeed, the characteristics of future generations. Over the past ten years, debates about this issue have recurred within the spheres of law, ethics and policy making on numerous occasions, from IVF to sperm utilization from comatose and subsequently deceased husbands, as in the Diane Blood case (*R.* v. *Human Fertilisation and Embryology Authority, ex p. Blood* 1997). This case was one of many that have provoked mixed reactions over whether individuals are entitled to make some claim of ownership over biological matter or, indeed, the specific coding that leads to the production of a particular type of species. Alternatively, one of the central controversies of mapping the human genome was the human genetic diversity project, codenamed the Vampire project. This project attempted to store the genetic data of peoples of indigenous populations, which have been steadily disappearing for many years. It was criticized for various reasons, one of which included a concern that the immortalization and potential commercial utilization of these data was an affront to the beliefs of some such nations (Dodson and Williamson 1999). Closely related to this issue are discussions about the ownership of genetic information generally and whether individuals or corporations can legitimately make claims over owning the information associated with genes (Spinello 2004). More recent instances of similar debates are the resurgent discourses on environmental concern, which invoke questions of ownership over nature in a broad and fundamental sense.

In what way do these two separate conversations on intellectual and biological property rights inform each other and how are they linked by our interest in the medicalization of cyberspace? Gordijn (2006) offers a useful indication when discussing the convergence of NBIC (nano, bio, info, cogno) technologies. When imagining the prospects of cognitive enhancement, Gordijn considers that

[i]f ... many different people were to share the possibility of being permanently connected to databases, the exclusiveness of possessing particular information would become relative, which in turn would reduce the uniqueness of those people. Implantation of brain-to-brain communication systems – which would 'wire up' different individuals to enable them to instantaneously exchange their conscious thoughts and experiences – could blur the borderline between the self and the cyberthink community. In the face of such mental wiring, how are one's own thoughts and experiences and life-history to be kept separate from those of others? And the borders between the real world and the virtual world would become increasingly blurred. As a result, it would become more and more difficult to determine one's own personal identity.

Here, Gordijn is interested in what might be described as the *hard* cyborg and alludes to our notion of biological property rights, where the biology of individuals is directly connected to technological systems. He is not referring to the '*soft* cyborg' (Zylinska 2005: 143), as one might describe the connection between people and their home computers, where intellectual property is dispersed across the Internet as part of the creative commons community. While Gordijn presents these prospects as problems or, at least, challenges, we are interested in considering how this expansion of property rights towards the biological could be seen similarly as a positive democratization of technology or, indeed, medical expertise. Perhaps contrary to his intentions, we consider that Gordijn's observation on the reduction of individual distinctiveness is a positive value in this context, as it confers a greater degree of freedom of expression and exploration. It also acknowledges the collaborative nature of creative expressions, either as cultural manifestations of body modification or as the emergence of credibility via user-generated reviews within the Internet.

In part, intellectual and biological property rights are also comparable in how the technology enables an ease and immediacy of choice over reproductive choice and, over the years there has been some crossover in analyses to strengthen this analogy. Indeed, the notion of the cyborg designates the relationship between biology and computerization – cybernetic organism. Overlaps are also evident in discussions about *cybersex,* again the interface of biology and cybernetics. Recall, again, from Chapter 6, the proposition that a rape took place in cyberspace, twice. Imaginations of cybersex have developed from text-based real-time (RT) interactions to full-blown teledildonic body-sex. Moreover, while many of these applications are not widespread, their prospect has become a prosthetic device of cybercultural imaginations. It is one of the narratives through which the future of humanity is imagined, where either sex is made sterile by its virtualization, or inhabitants of a sophisticated technological civilization no longer deem sexual desire valuable. Again, one can consider the Ron's Angels case as an indication of this prospect, where reproduction is reduced to liberal, disembodied actions of procreators rather than parents.

The co-development of these leisurely technologies takes place amid the clinical aspects of reproduction, health and artificial insemination, as an integral part of medicalized cyberspace. Moreover, there is an overlap between the conceptual language through which one discusses cybersexual freedom and the regulation of (cyber)sexualized bodies. Yet the questions over disembodiment that have emerged from such activities are less interesting than the way in which cybersexuality can be understood as a process of reproduction and/or hyper-contraception. Cybersex is simultaneously a refuge for the lonely, the promiscuous, the cautious, the afraid and the curious. Importantly, it is not cybersex at all, it is cyber-reproduction: the creation of newborns through multi-networked machines. As Kember (1999: 29) argues, 'medicine can now simulate, capture and seemingly recreate the human body in cyberspace, and this, for me, is another facet of autonomous reproduction'. Moreover, with the assistance of an interactive virtual reality device, cybersex can be a physiological process leading to actual procreation by the insertion of semen via an artificial penis (Zhai 1997). People may choose to reproduce through engaging in a simulated sexual experience, while only engaging in intercourse within a virtual world. Alternatively, 'the biological process of procreation can be carried out in addition to the fulfilment of the sexual desire and emotional needs of both partners' (ibid.) as a couple who may reproduce remotely. These possibilities encourage the consideration of how one understands reproductive rights and the conceptualization of bodies, reproduction and health within such techno-medical contexts. In short, they invite us to ask what matters about reproductive liberty when a crucial aspect of the embodied practice becomes reconstituted via technology.

Viagra, spam and cyberpharmacies

As we indicated at the outset of this chapter, our intention is to work towards contextualizing some of the legal concerns about cybermedicine, rather than to deal in depth with the specific legal issues it presents. This has been done elsewhere by a number of authors (see Terry 1999; Ward 2003). Thus far, we have identified that there is common ground in the languages surrounding intellectual and biological property rights and that this should inform our interpretation of the debate about medicalized cyberspace. There remain considerable uncertainties about who owns online communities, what legal claims can be made over them and, by implication, who should regulate them. A significant component of this debate within medicine has been the regulation of products and treatments that are delivered over the Internet.

Concerns about the medicalizing effects of industries that use the media to promote pharmaceutical solutions to health-related conditions have been evident since the 1970s. Stimson (1975: 159) notes that 'the advertising of psychotropic drugs defines certain types of people as potentially in need of such drugs and defines certain life events and situations as illness'. Also, Conrad and Schneider (1980) discuss Ritalin and methadone as instances of medicalization via the pharmaceutical industry.[2] Nevertheless, one of the most recent visible symbols of the emergent procreative choices we have discussed is a prosthetic device that was made notorious by online commerce: *Viagra*. An icon of our present-day future, this cyberspatial wonder drug is consumed daily by email(male) spam and health sites (Eysenbach 1999). Via this new technology, men are repeatedly informed of their inadequacy in a brave new world where procreative capacity and sexual prowess must, or at least should, be purchased.

Viagra (sildenafil citrate) is the perpetually new male anti-contraceptive, a means to greater virility, while the male contraceptive pill remains unattainable.[3] As a paradigm of the cybersex industry, its emergence elicited various responses, from claims that it reinforces patriarchal values by defining sexuality via the male erection, to intricate studies that suggest the technology cannot be treated in any general sense, since neither erectile dysfunction nor erectile functioning are universal concepts (Potts 2004). Viagra has been a central part of recent discussions about the regulation of online pharmacies. An integral part of Viagra's development occurred via the Internet, which emerged at the height of the dotcom boom.

Marshall notes that 'hundreds of internet sites emerged which offered online prescriptions and home delivery' (2002: 133). Moreover, Kahan *et al.* (2000: 921) claim that it is 'by far the most commonly prescribed online drug'.[4]

The circulation of pharmaceutical products via the Internet is one of the most visible and far-reaching aspects of how cyberspace has become medicalized. Indeed, Vares and Braun (2006) note that Viagra was one of the top ten spam topics in 2003, and Loe (2004) documents the range of strategies that were used to market this product. In the context of this marketing, Conrad identifies that it is crucial to understand the 'impact of the Internet' (2005: 12) in constituting contemporary medicalization debates.

Our consideration of this case offers a further parameter to our analysis, which is closely connected to the discussion about whether online environments can be regulated by the medical profession. In this case, the worldwide distribution of pharmaceuticals – particularly those that perform a non-therapeutic or 'lifestyle' function – crystallizes the challenges raised by the redrawing of boundaries that the Internet provokes. It constitutes an arena where fears over the expansion of (cyber)medical liberty operate under an assumption that commercial factors *will* shape the nature of such liberty and that this will undermine human flourishing.[5] These views are shared by a number of scholars of Viagra. For instance, Tiefer (2006: 274) notes that Viagra 'participates in the evolving consumerist and Internet technologies of sexual recreation and sexual self-determination for privileged men and women of the "sex and the city" and baby boom "you can have it all" and "positive aging" generations.' Also, Morgentaler (2003) describes the myth that Viagra is a quick fix to complex sexual problems within relationships. An integral component of this process of 'corporatized medicalization' (Conrad 2005: 11) is its tendency to utilize gendered technologies as a 'strategy for defining problems and promoting medical solutions, both exploring and reinforcing gender boundaries' (ibid.). This is also why an analysis of Viagra is of particular concern to us. This so-called wonder drug corresponds with the wonder expressed about the Internet, an imaginative series of possibilities and experience enabled by an arrangement of technics that arises out of the inadequacy of previous modes of communication.

The types of websites that distribute medical products, particularly pharmaceuticals, vary considerably, and many do not fit neatly into a category that might be described as an online pharmacy. Such websites play an active part in offering consultation, advice, information and medication that accommodates the range of interests of online users. The perceived dangers of this dimension of cybermedicine are extensive. For instance, Burgermeister (2004: 603) notes that the United Nations' reaction to drugs sold on the Internet characterizes the phenomenon as 'an increasing risk to people's health'. The UN report makes special reference to Viagra, though the observation occurs many years after the product first drew attention over its potential to be distributed online: 'Surfing the internet illustrates the bigger problem. Sildenafil can be obtained by anyone who wants it' (*The Lancet* 1998: 751). This editorial from *The Lancet* is also exemplary of the continual overlap between cybermedicine and cybrersexuality that our overall analysis attends to:

The internet, irregular supplies apart, provides access to a mix of information on sildenafil from the responsible material put up on the US Food and Drug Administration and Pfizer websites to a Viagra message board with signposting to pornographic material.

(ibid.)

An additional problem facing the regulation of online pharmaceuticals is the legal determination of geographical *boundaries* and the uncertainty over how domestic law should treat transgressions of these boundaries. For instance, Spurgeon (2003) explores the relationship between US and Canadian law on the regulation of medication over the importing of cheap drugs to the United States from Canada. While the United States has a fiscal and regulatory interest in taking action over such transgressions, questions arise as to whether it is reasonable to prosecute individuals who undertake such decisions, owing to the absence of adequate and affordable health care. In this sense, instituting criminal action against such vulnerable groups would be contrary to principles of social welfare, particularly when so many are senior citizens (Cohen 2004). To comprehend the range of civil liability issues that are at stake over the regulation of cyberpharmacies, Kahan *et al.* (2000) offer a number of categories: confidentiality, medical malpractice, physician licensure, product liability and class action. For each of these, there is considerable uncertainty about how they should be addressed in the context of an online substance. However, there is a general sense that medical practice is being transformed as the Internet develops.

Nevertheless, the appeal of cybermedicine has ideological roots that are deeply entrenched in the broader empancipatory aspirations for the Internet. For example, in the United Kingdom such ideas were reflected in various white papers that emphasized the importance of patient empowerment and the 'patient's active involvement in discussions about their health' (Hardey 1999: 821). They are reflected, too, in attempts to prepare the pharmacy profession for the utilization of information and communications technologies (Department of Health 2003). There is, of course, also an efficiency benefit, which raises other questions. For instance, one might argue that the process of democratizing medical knowledge also shifts legal and moral responsibilities of health care towards the patient and away from the profession.

The questions we posed at the beginning of this chapter, in particular whether there is a need to consider the notion of a virtual exceptionalism when discussing the practice of medicine in cyberspace, should be answered positively. The ethics of body trafficking online is radically altered by the expansion of biological property rights. The regulation of cybermedical practices over the Internet cannot rely on a top-down, principled implementation of ethics, as one might expect from professional codes of ethics, since the notion of the medical expert in cyberspace is diverse. Moreover, the legal boundaries of medical regulation imply the need to consider more carefully the global character of health care and the rise of medical tourism.

The end of medical history and the last prosthesis

The medicalization of cyberspace is, thus, a watershed for how we make sense of cyberspace and medicine. In this context, Viagra constitutes the end of medical history, as it signals a conceptual shift into the terrain of lifestyled reproductive freedom. It constitutes the 'escape velocity' (Dery 1996) of biotechnology, as it traverses into the real of the posthuman. Its prosthetic character – as a replacement for something lost, or which might never have been – occurs within a biopolitical frame that has been shaped by Fukuyama's elaboration on the end of history (2002). Fukuyama's trajectory from political economy to biopolitics reinforces the idea that medicalization is at a precipice – facing biomedicalization – where critical boundaries are transgressed by the decentralization of biomedical decision making.

Indeed, a reading of Fukuyama's development from the 'end of history' towards the end of bioethics (Fukuyama and Furger 2007) reveals the broader depth of these issues. As he notes, the era of biotechnology has the potential to lead to the abolition of 'human beings as such' and to usher in 'a new posthuman history'. Fukuyama (1999) also reminds us, again, of the centrality of connections between information and biology, which he characterizes as the 'twin revolutions' (1999: 18). Our reading of Viagra as the last prosthesis tells us of the cultural character of biological modifications and the medicalization of cyberspace. Our claim is not that other prostheses will cease to exist, but that Viagra signifies the shift in how prostheses will look and become part of a lifestyled culture. Thus, the concept of the last prosthesis conveys the cessation of artefacts as prosthesis, as technology becomes symbiotic with biology. Viagra's depiction of a simulated substance underneath the skin suggests the final realm of the exterior prosthesis, as technology becomes part of biology, infecting it with thousands of nano devices. This last prosthesis, at the interface with the first and original prosthesis, the body, indicates the promise of 'better choices to come' (Marshall 2002).[6]

8   The online Pro-Ana movement

In this chapter, we examine the formation of particular and distinctive cyber-medical communities that are deemed, in some ways, to be instances of harmful body modification. We take up this discussion via an examination of websites that are collectively recognized as Pro-Anorexia communities; Pro-Anorexia has been defined as promoting a 'managed approach to anorexia and has sought to re-define it outside medical or other professional discourses' (Fox *et al*. 2005b: 945). This is a particularly interesting case from which to discuss the moral and ethical implications of cybermedical connections, not least because it has been one of the few instances of a cybermedical issue where websites have been considered harmful enough to be removed from the World Wide Web by Internet service providers. Moreover, its online presence has prompted a response of moral panic from the media and particular agencies, who have utilized the case in wider debates about the nature and treatment of anorexia (Ferreday 2003).

We consider how the obvious unification that these net users are seeking may inform our understanding of such complex bodily 'disorders'. Undertaking this task means exploring the ontology of these cyberspaces, the realities that are created within, through and beyond them. How, for example, are they utilized in wider discourse on eating disorders and the body? The way we understand the ontological structure of these cyberspaces determines how particular realities can exist within it (Heim 1993). Hence, we explore the structure, nature and distinctive features of these cyberspaces, in relation to the social construction and experiences of anorexia. In Chapter 9, we shall consider how Pro-Ana may be considered in broader discussions about feminism, digital culture and bioethics.

Pro-Ana environments

Pro-Ana has emerged primarily through a variety of Internet-based Web sites and networks (see Brown 2001; Reaves 2001; Taylor 2002; Chesley *et al*. 2003) rather than in real-time support groups. Many of these sites 'provide specific instructions for initiating and maintaining bulimia and anorexia' (Chesley *et al*. 2003: 123) and include bulletin boards, weblogs, discussion forums and chat rooms where users can exchange messages and interact with others. Diaries, biographies and stories have also become a common feature of these forums, with website owners and visitors posting reports on their calorie intake and writing about their experiences relating to their eating disorders, including hospitalization, recovery, and so on. The content of these Internet sites varies greatly: one can find support from others experiencing an eating disorder or, more controversially, garner information and advice on the way to develop an eating disorder or conceal it from others. Some sites adopt more obvious Pro-Ana identities within their titles (for examples, see Anagurls live journal, anorexic beauty, anorexic nation, Go Ana, Love it to death, worship in vain, starving for perfection, wasting away on the web, dying to be thin).

Concerns have been raised about the potentially harmful interactions that may take place in these environments, including online competitions to become the best anorexic. On some websites, tips and tricks relating to the 'practice' of anorexia (see Warin 2004; Rich 2006) are shared between anorexics. Other studies have revealed that these environments are also used 'for dispensing information related to nutrition, and techniques to lose or gain weight' (Chesley *et al.* 2003: 123), ways to hide or avoid food, and methods to conceal anorexia from significant others. In addition, many of them contain what are called 'thinspiration' galleries that show pictures of emaciated young women, or famously thin models and actresses (see Ferreday 2003).

A handful of recent studies have highlighted the reaction from media and other agencies to these networks. For example, Ferreday (2003: 288) argues that the popular press tend to report 'disgust' over the portrayal of the anorexic body and 'by producing a physical sensation of revulsion, the anorexic body breaks down the distinction between the healthy subject and the abject other' (ibid.). Many of these websites focus on anorexia rather than bulimia, or use Pro-Ana to represent both anorexia and bulimia. Henceforth, we shall therefore refer to these websites collectively as 'Pro-Ana'.

The Pro-Ana movement is a particularly challenging case for medical ethics and raises a number of issues that connect with broader discussions within cyberfeminist bioethics. The collective removal of these websites from the Internet was partly in response to concerns voiced by the media (Ferreday 2003: 288), medical communities, and families and friends of those with eating disorders. In 2001, ANAD (Anorexia Nervosa and Associated Disorders), an American eating disorder advocacy group, called for servers to take down what were considered particularly harmful Pro-Ana sites. Subsequently, some Internet servers stopped hosting these websites. Pro-Ana material continued to be made available online through other means, and the development of Web 2.0 has since provided opportunities for Pro-Ana members to communicate in more sophisticated and unregulated ways, including, for example, the use of video diaries.

As Pollack (2003: 246–247) reports, there are now a number of groups opposing these websites, including S.C.a.R.E.D. (Support, Concern, and Resources for Eating Disorders) and S.P.A.P. (Stopping Pro-Anorexia Promotion), which have their own websites, hoping to 'raise awareness' about the Pro-Ana movement and prevent people from visiting and using their Web material. Recent studies on Pro-Ana websites (Dias 2003; Ferreday 2003; Pollack 2003) have revealed that the media and other agencies often use a discourse of sensationalism:

> [T]he articles often demonize the creators of the sites, blaming the 'anorex-ics' infamous defensive talents' (Time.com, 2001), 'misguided ideas' (CWK network – Sodano, 2002) and group 'delusion' (Salon.com – Brown, 2001) for the seemingly infectious spread of eating disorders.
>
> (Pollack 2003: 246)

Moreover, many of the concerns raised about Pro-Ana have focused on particular types of website that offer more extreme advice and material on severe weight loss. Other Pro-Ana sites offer what might be considered as more temperate views around anorexia and may actually offer support to recovery.[1] As with these other authors, rather than dismiss these spaces as dangerous and of no value, our inter-est is to understand the multiple discourses that are present in Pro-Ana networks. Within these environments, cybermedical discourses reconstitute anorexia and the anorexic body in multiple and, sometimes, competing ways.

The emergence of these types of communities within an expanding and ubiq-uitous presence of networked information has led to a moral panic associated with concerns about freedom of knowledge. Pro-Ana brings forth very distinct con-cerns about the governance of alternative health knowledge. This sensationalist response to these digital environments draws upon technological determinism (see Kitchin 1998) and positions Pro-Ana in some imagined future where it has the capacity to sway others into an incredibly complex health condition. Young women are positioned as potentially vulnerable and prone to being swayed by Pro-Ana; consider the following online media article:

> The problem, of course, is that most of the minds visiting these sites are not exactly in peak psychological condition. And many of the sites, with their rosy color schemes and celebrity slide shows, are designed to appeal to the most vulnerable population. This labored enthusiasm serves as a red flag to eating disorders educators like Meehan. 'One of the primary goals of anorex-ics is to persuade others that they are perfectly fine, and that they have the right to lead their lives however they see fit,' says Meehan. 'And one of the ways of doing that is to find other people who are achieving those goals – so these web sites provide not only reinforcement, along with a forum for exchanging and picking up tips.'
>
> (Reaves 2001)

In this vein, the reaction to Pro-Ana reflects Hall's (1996: 167) claim that, far from embodying Haraway's cyborg ideologies, 'cyberspace is creating god-desses and ogres, not cyborgs'. Like Dias (2003) we remain concerned that over-simplistic and reductive notions of complex online interactions may only serve to further pathologize eating disorders (see Rich and Evans 2005). As a result, we might be 'left with the impression that the problem lies here, in these individual women and the "outrageous" practices that they endorse via the Internet' (Dias 2003: 37). Such interpretations tend to reify typical aetiologies of eating disorders that draw upon the ideas that the person is emotionally unbalanced, needy, a perfectionist, desires control or has cognitive distortions (see Cogan 1999: 231).[2] Dias (2003) goes on to suggest that many of the voices and experiences of those actually using these sites have tended to be silenced by these sensationalist discourses.

While we have no wish to promote discourses which propel individuals towards serious ill health and, in some cases, near-death, one cannot dismiss these spaces as wholly dangerous. The challenge ahead involves an interpretation of these spaces, rather than treating them simplistically as dangerous. In many ways, they are political sites that reveal a great deal about how discourses of gender, technology and the body limit the construction of particular body narratives. Pro-Ana sites may have harmful and negative features, but to assume that such networks are a reflection of a group of troubled young women who want to harm themselves and others through the promotion of eating disorders would be to oversimplify an extremely complex condition related to the body, health and food. Rather, it is necessary to consider the complex ways that women are making sense of their bodies, health and 'self' in these spaces and ask what type of cyberpolitics is invoked.

Pro-Ana voices

In what follows, we draw on open-access websites to explore the Pro-Ana movement in two ways. First, data are taken from a Pro-Ana blog to explore the various ways in which young women are engaging with pro-anorexia. Data extracted from this blog are referenced as: (anonymous user, Pro-Ana blog). Second, we draw upon online debates between Pro-Ana users and other anorectics who were critical of Pro-Ana websites. This public dialogue was accessed via an eating disorders (non-'Pro-Ana') support blog. Data extracts from this blog are referenced as: (anonymous user, ED support blog).

Following Bruckman (2001), we accessed websites that were publicly archived but did not require a password to gain access. Accordingly, while it was not necessary to obtain informed consent, we have removed all the URL links, names and usernames (pseudonyms used when leaving a message) as a way of protecting the confidentiality of the blog and its members.[3] We did not join any of these blogs as members, or post any messages, but downloaded and analysed archives from the Pro-Ana site over a six-month period during 2005, and for the eating disorders blog archives over a six-month period in 2003, which featured the Pro-Ana debate. These archives featured messages from a wide variety of users, some of whom visited the blog regularly.

The politics of Pro-Ana

Perhaps unsurprisingly, cyberspace is being utilized by Pro-Ana users as a way of networking and finding support from others – a position that contrasts greatly with discourses that position Pro-Ana sites as subversive (Pollack, 2003). The importance of these networks must be considered in the wider context, where eating disorders are extremely complex, damaging and isolating conditions, but often remain grossly unreported (Walstrom 2000: 762). In many ways, Pro-Ana occupies a political space, mobilizing digital environments to make public body-narratives that might otherwise go untold (Dias 2003). That these narratives occur in digital contexts is no coincidence. Indeed, part of our interest in cyber-communities and eating disorders stems from work elsewhere where we have highlighted that young women tend to experience a lack of 'relatedness' (Warin 2003: 89) between the experiences they wanted to voice to significant others and the stories they actually told (see Rich and Evans 2005). As was discussed in Chapter 5, embodied, painful and often chaotic narratives of illness can be silenced by wider medicalized discourses of health and illness. The exchange of alternative body-narratives around eating disorders resonates with the sort of cyborg presence in Haraway's manifesto: 'Cyborg writing is about the power to survive, not on the basis of original innocence, but on the basis of seizing the tools to mark the world that marked them as other' (1991: 175).

As with others, our interest is to consider how discourses of anorexia within cyberspace may offer alternative 'explanatory models' (Fox *et al.* 2005b) of the body, health and illness. Like other eating disorders, anorexia is an extremely complex condition variously understood and much debated across the disciplines of psychiatry, medicine, psychology, biology, sociology and epidemiology. Our intention is not to understate the sophistication of the perspectives that abound within these fields (see Lask and Bryant-Waugh 2000). Thus, discourses of anorexia draw upon various frameworks of understanding, from biomedical models that evaluate anorexia as a disease with an underlying 'organic' cause (Urwin *et al.* 2002) to those that emphasize the psychological, social and cultural roots of eating disorders. Fox *et al.* (2005b: 945) suggest that while the causal explanations and treatment recommendations vary across these western models, they differ from Pro-Ana in that they 'all serve as explanatory models of a disease to be remedied'.

Our interest in the formation of Pro-Ana networks connects with research exploring how anorexia comes to be managed as both an identity and an illness (Rich 2006). These tensions emerge at the intersection of competing discourses around what constitutes anorexia and how, if at all, it should be managed or treated. Young women with anorexia often find that significant others in their lives tend to position themselves against discourses of disease. In doing so, a 'restitution narrative' (Frank 1995) is often invoked when trying to offer support and make sense of these conditions (Rich 2006). This narrative is grounded in the ideals associated with treatment and reparation. It centres on what will be done to restore the body to its former state before illness, or towards medically defined standards of the healthy body. This narrative centres on the expectation that individuals should make rational choices to return to normal health, or indeed achieve desired states of health, despite the contested nature of these concepts. The effect of this is that 'the anorexic's determination to starve in the face of such abundance is essentially seen as irrational' (Draper 2000: 129). The tensions caused around the social construction of anorexia were a regular feature of the topics of discussion within the blogs we examined:

> also my mum and sister are ALWAYS on my case, checking on me and force feeding me and crying when I won't eat.
>
> (Anonymous user, Pro-Ana blog)

> What sucked is no one wanted to listen to my problems, no one cared.
>
> (Anonymous user, Pro-Ana blog)

> I wish I had one friend who would understand me and I could talk to about my problems ... but I don't ... none of my friends would understand.
>
> (Anonymous user, Pro-Ana blog)

Online environments are utilized to manage the forms of 'discursive constraint' (Ronai 1997: 125, cited in Cordell and Ronai 1999) they experience in other contexts, wherein their 'behaviour is constrained by the threat of having a negative category applied to ... herself. These categories are disseminated throughout society so effectively that they take on a taken for granted or given quality' (Ronai 1997: 125).

Within these medicalized and psychiatrized discourses (Harwood 2006), anorexia becomes defined as a negative social position through which to establish a sense of self, implicitly working to persuade someone to return to 'normal/healthy' weight. It constrains the discourse that these young women can apply to their self (Cordell and Ronai 1999), reducing the available subjectivities to positions of irrationality or pathology. Anorexia becomes positioned as 'other' through these discourses, as the 'body that "has" difference' (Ferreday 2003: 277). As Komesaroff (1995: 4) observes, where common social practices are formulated in the language of pathology, the possibility of a moral evaluation of them is introduced. To this end, 'otherness' is conceived of as 'different' or even 'deviant' and propels many of these users to keep returning Pro-Ana environments:

> I swore never to come on here again, but there is no place like home. I kept saying to myself, 'You are fine. Even if you have gained some weight, you are still considered underweight. I'll just give my mum a break and be *normal.*' Well, I can be normal to her and perfect to me.
>
> (Anonymous user, Pro-Ana blog; our emphasis)

The narratives made public in these Web spaces reveal how many of these young women were managing anorexia as both an identity and an illness category that may lead to processes of 'subjectivisation' (Foucault 1996: 472) (see

Rich and Evans 2005). What are seemingly peculiar networks seem to occupy a more obvious presence when considered against this context of wider patholo-gization of anorexia:

> They [Internet sites] are the ONLY form of consistency and true support. You would not believe how many of us spend hours talking to the younger ones about the consequences and yeah about death. These kids learn fast and no one holds back. Once the talking about the eating disorder is talked about the real pain comes through. The thought of you shutting my support down like, when I just read some of the posts the first thing that popped into my head was, I can kill myself.
>
> (Anonymous user, ED support blog)

> The site I belong to could be classified as proana but they offer everything from recovery to those 12 year olds begging for advice on how to become an anorexic. Most of all it is a place for people to vent about every issue you could image. It frightens the hell out of me that people like you go around and take away our rights to freedom of speech.
>
> (Anonymous user, ED support blog)

> It's a very isolating illness which is why so many people find these boards helpful – they can't talk about it with many people in their 'real life'.
>
> (Anonymous user, ED support blog)

These cyberspaces, as one user suggests, become 'a place to talk about ED, get support, and share stories. You can say whatever you want here'. Dias (2003) refers to this as a 'sanctuary' for many anorexics. In some cases, users visit these spaces because they provide a context where they can 'discuss their problems in a sympa-thetic and non-censorious environment that may be lacking in their everyday lives' (Ferreday 2003: 284). These digital connections provide considerable appeal:

> You don't realize how close people become, how helpful people are when it comes to helping others out when they don't want to puke anymore. They are the ONLY form of consistency and true support.
>
> (Anonymous user, ED support group)

Within these environments, contradictory, multiple experiences form part of the fabric of regular interaction. These environments were different from those pro-vided by other eating disorder support groups, because the network did not take some collective view that anorexia was a disease to be fixed. Some users inti-mated that this meant they could talk more openly about the contradictory feelings they had about their bodies and anorexia, without fear of reproach:

> People need to go where they feel that they can openly talk about their ED, thoughts and behaviours. It's a process where people need to know that yeah

they have the choice to go to therapy and be honest in order to recover. ... People don't always need to be told that what they are doing is wrong, they know. They need to explore and express.

(Anonymous user, ED support blog)

The freedom to express desires and pleasurable aspects of anorexia confers value to these spaces, which, rather than suggesting that they should be removed, raises questions about how similar spaces might be enabled elsewhere.

I think it is easier to deal with a problem if it is out in the open.

(Anonymous user, ED support blog)

I myself have come to the conclusion, after years on denial about even having one [a problem], that I like it and its like a part of me.

(Anonymous user, Pro-Ana blog)

I'll admit I tried to recover before and even left this community for a while, and I just felt very lost. I also felt like i was denying a part of myself, trying to become something I wasn't cut out to be. I relapsed but not after months of struggles trying to become 'normal' and 'healthy' again.

(Anonymous user, Pro-Ana blog)

From the perspective of such cyborg feminists as Haraway (1991), these narratives resonate with the cyborg: the shift towards the fluid, situatedness, and embracing of contradictory subjectivities – in this case, of feeling empowered by anorexia yet also having an awareness of its destructive nature:

I personally think that when you are in the depths of your ED [eating disorder], it is extremely difficult to know if you want to recover or not. Anorexia is everything to you. If you asked me if I wanted to give up the anorexia back then, I would have said no. But still something deep down inside of me (that little bit of healthy brain that I still had) knew that something wasn't right. Why would something that was supposed to make me feel so good about myself and my body make me feel so bad about myself and my body? Surely there had to be another way to live. I wasn't living ... I was dying. I lost so much more than weight. I lost my perfect grades, I lost so many friends, I lost my passion for things I liked, and most of all I lost myself and everything that defined me. I became the anorexia. Anorexia was my 'life'. I didn't choose to 'give up' anorexia. Rather, I chose to gain life, which means gaining weight, gaining self esteem, gaining self respect, and so much more.

(Anonymous user, ED support blog)

I am a member of some pro ana sites as well as some recovery sites. ... Yes there are definitely areas of the sites that are not for my own good but I have a hard time balancing the idea with having no availability to that support that I feel from them.

(Anonymous user, ED support blog)

Far from propelling *all* women into further destructive relationships with anorexia, the Pro-Ana cyber-communities are appropriated in different ways by different users. Indeed, for some, they provide a context in which being able to talk about the ambivalence of anorexia forms a productive part of the process of recovery:

> You would not believe how people have actually left for recovery. When you can't trust many people and then you finally find that source of expression you find relief, you find hope, you find understanding, you find friends. Right now I'm having a massive heart attack as I write this because you are taking away the hope I have. It's incredible how much relief you feel when you have found someone who has similar experiences as you. You find that hope.
>
> (Anonymous user, ED support blog)

> I have never had to hide my behaviors or trick my doctor. When someone is forced into recovery, they feel as if you are taking their control away, which makes them want to continue the behaviors even more, and when they get out they are even more determined than when they went in. I am not anti recovery, I just think a person has to want to recover for it to be of any help for them.
>
> (Anonymous user, ED support blog)

> All you anti-Pro-Anas are just pathetic. Why try to stop people from expressing their opinions?! Pro ana websites are here to help people and give support no matter what they want to do. What your saying is that if you met an anorexic who had no intention of trying to recover they are wr0ng and they should be forced into recovery. Most of these websites actually help people recover by offering them support. Everyone there cares for each other and just wants each other to be happy and who are you to meddle with this?! Are you saying that you would rather have people with eating disorders lonely until they finally see your point of view?! Cos it sounds like it when your trying to split up whole Web communities because [they] try to help each other in whatever decision they make.
>
> (Anonymous user, ED support blog)

As Dias (2003:1) reminds us, Pro-Ana spaces highlight the politicization of body narratives: 'Just as the body is a site of struggle (and resistance), so too there are struggles over where and how women's stories of their body can be told.' As one of the few studies on these spaces, Dias' work alludes to the importance of these spaces for women to find sanctuary and construct particular stories of their anorexia. In these digital environments, young women can – and do – talk about dietary practices, emotions, pain and experiences that they feel may elsewhere be pathologized or silenced. The reinscription of anorexia via Pro-Ana in some ways acts as a form of narrative resistance to dichotomies around health/ill health (Ronai 1994). Rather than constructing anorectics as irrational, seeking attention or abnormal, some Pro-Ana users construct alternatives narratives of superiority and control:

> Those who visit Pro-Ana sites are not mindless automatons who can be brainwashed just from seeing what is on the site. Anorexia takes a lot of determination, and if someone is bent on being anorexic they will find a way, with or without the Internet.
>
> (Anonymous user, ED support blog)

Disciplined dietary restraint is used as a way of demonstrating self-control, autonomy and individuality, and achieving recognition from others. Some sites associated with the Pro-Ana movement also sell Pro-Ana or Pro-Mia 'identity' bracelets:

> Hey Guys and Girls, there is a new craze which is going to sweep over ... we HAVE to be first and establish it as a sign of Ana/Mias' presence ... go to www.oafcharm.co.uk and order one!! Black is for strength – we should each get one as a sign of our control and strength in what we do.
>
> (Anonymous user, Pro-Ana blog)

Many of our observations thus far resonate with those of the handful of authors (Ferreday 2003; Dias 2003; Pollack 2003) who have explored eating disorders in online environments. In building on these studies, we wish to connect some of these insights with our thesis on a cybermedicalization and how this mediates Pro-Ana environments.

Pro-Ana and cybermedicalization

> I choose to be thin because it's the only way I am happy with myself. I support it, and we have the right to live the way we want to live. I hate that people try to single us out. Are they jelous? Why are they over concerned about our self-image. ... OUR choices?!!! I am not sickly, I just want to be thin. There is NOTHING wrong with that.
>
> (Anonymous user, ED support group)

The notion that anorexia becomes 'managed as both an illness and identity' (Rich 2006) category is particularly evident in Pro-Ana's contradictory engagement with processes of cybermedicalization. Many of the Pro-Ana narratives, like the one above, constitute anorexia as a lifestyle choice. A cursory reading of these comments might lead to all sorts of ethical concerns about people 'choosing' to undertake extreme weight loss. Indeed, it would too simplistic to explain these comments via the usual discourse of young women being swayed by popular culture and media imagery of thin celebrities. However, the narratives of Pro-Ana users also indicate a response to the pathological stereotypes of anorexia as a media-driven slimmer's disease. Although the intention in Pro-Ana may be to 'subvert medical models of anorexia' (Ferreday 2003: 285), as explored in Chapter 5, there are also occasions where medicalized discourses are drawn upon simultaneously. This was particularly the case when the term 'wannabes' was used in online discussions. Wannabes was a label denoting young women who had engaged with anorexic behaviours but as a lifestyle choice, or had promoted anorexia as a glamorous lifestyle:

> [O]n the site I belong too, they are called 'wannabe's.' Girls come to the site asking how they develop an ED.
>
> (Anonymous user, ED support blog).

> [W]hen I visit a Pro-Ana site and see a 15 year old girl saying 'oh wow, I'm going to give all these tips and tricks to my friends who want to be ana' ... well, I'm afraid that I AM going to be just a little bit critical in my response.
>
> (Anonymous user, ED support blog).

> I have a lot of time for people who are doing it rough, but not a lot for those who look on it as a 'glamour' lifestyle and promote it to their friends.
>
> (Anonymous user, ED support blog).

Many of the users distinguish between anorectics and 'wannabes', but, rather ironically, do so by drawing upon a medicalized discourse of a kind that in other interactions they revoke:

> I guess my point is that not all proana sites are bad. ... I can tell you though i have been to some who full on promote anorexia as a lifestyle, its not its a *disease* and people need to understand that.
>
> (Anonymous user, ED support blog)

In accounts like these, rather than constructing a dichotomy between anorexia as identity (lifestyle choice) and illness (disease category) (Rich 2006), one can see the utilization of explanatory frameworks of disease to legitimize a contradictory 'identity'. This is a particularly complex process, although Malson's (1998: 152) research on the social psychology of anorexia nervosa is instructive here. She argues that accounting for anorexia in terms of a social pressure to be thin – to live up to an 'ideal' – undermines one's position as a unitary, self-directed individual. Constructing oneself as a unitary, rational individual is a critical feature of some of the narratives that defend the right to choose anorexia as a 'lifestyle' that should be managed rather than treated. Thus, Pro-Ana users face the difficult task of constructing a narrative that counters the idea that they are swayed by social process while also challenging the idea that anorexia is a disease to be remedied. Connections and contestations between 'wannabes' and 'anorexics' therefore take on a hypertextuality, both linked and distanced via similar discourses. By emphasizing a medicalized discourse, Pro-Ana users are able to stress the seriousness of their condition as a way of distinguishing themselves from wannabes.

> All i want to say basically is that anorexia nervosa as been around a long long time b4 the internet was even dreamed of so i dont blame blame pro sites what i do blame is the wannabie teenages who thinks its cool to have this illness like some kinda statement i say ILLNESS because that is what it is u cant become anorexic you cant make your self anorexic its going to take more than a few pics of skinny gals on a trigger site for you to starve yourself to the point of death and distroy your family and be in pain physically and mentaly so excuse me but all u teenie wana bes make me quite sick and mad if u get rid of pro ana then u will not get rid of anorexia.
>
> (Anonymous user, ED support blog)

> I know you do not agree with the content anyway, but our site does recognize that it is a disorder not a lifestyle and we do not advocate it as a lifestyle.
>
> (Anonymous user, ED support blog)

> Please point me in the direction of a single MEDICALLY APPROVED article on the Web that advocates a Pro-ED stance – I'd be interested to read it. In my extensive research into the Pro-ED mindset, I have yet to discover ANYONE in the medical profession who agrees with pro-ED.
>
> (Anonymous user, ED support blog).

> Anorexia is not a diet nor the easy way out, its a disease, its like cancer and AIDS. So i suggest you get some common sense and think before you put up posts.
>
> (Anonymous user, ED support blog)

Thus, although Pro-Ana may attempt to challenge biomedical models of anorexia, it may also be infused with confounding limitations arising from cybermedical processes. As Pollack (2003: 249) suggests, engaging with this sort of 'reverse discourse' may be relevant to the Pro-Ana community by reappropriating medicalized language: 'from oppressive to agentic, the pro-eating disorders subject's public attempts to embrace the disorder can be seen as a complex political action' (ibid.).

Pro-Ana bodies

Within the so-called 'thinspiration' galleries, the body is not only present in this observable form, but comes to be reconstituted via body narratives. Body modification narratives were revealed in interactions where Pro-Ana users exchanged tips and experiences of engaging with anorexic practices (see Warin 2004: 101). Descriptions of these methods tended to draw upon the visceral features of these experiences:

Does anyone know of anyway to get rid of dizziness and nausea without eating? I tried drinking water but it only made it worse.

(Anonymous user, Pro-Ana blog)

Two days ago i stopped eating and i held out until just a couple minutes ago when i ate an apple and some doritos!!! i feel so disgusting. can someone help me? i need tips on how to just say no to food.

(Anonymous user, Pro-Ana blog)

Is there anyway to trick a doctor into thinking that you are almost fully recovered and that you dont have an eating disorder anymore? REPLY: i haven't been hospitalized cause i've only purged a couple of times and im not that skinny lol but i do know that a dentist can tell if you throw up becuase it deteriorates the enamel on your teeth so just be careful if you have a dentist appointment soon. i know that wasnt really your question but i figured any tips i could give can help for the future :) luv ya.

(Anonymous user, Pro-Ana blog)

Any who ... have any of you guys tried zantrex-3? I just got some and they make me so sick and grouchy! ... (aleast to sick to eat) but I was just wondering if they have really worked, also I got slim mints ???? any thoughts about those?

(Anonymous user, Pro-Ana blog)

Concerns continue to be raised about the advice available on these websites for extreme weight loss and body modification. For example, Fox *et al.* (2005b) report the use of multi-vitamins to supplement a restricted anorectic diet; encouragement in the form of thinspiration and discussions of the use of weight-loss pharmaceuticals. Other materials on Pro-Ana sites include technique and nutrition sections that prescribe habits and practices for weight loss (Chesley *et al.* 2003). These networks are also utilized for the sharing of what are termed 'anorexic tricks' (Warin 2002: 132) to either develop anorexia or conceal it from others.

The presence of these narratives in cyberspace may, in this sense, act as a technique for constructing a particular subjectivity and form of embodiment. Indeed, as Stryker notes, 'Flesh is not often visually performative in cyberspace, and yet the subjects communicating there are inextricably caught up in other interactive webs where flesh matters a great deal' (2000: 594–595). Stryker's claims seem even more poignant now, given the inherently rich content of many Web 2.0 spaces, such as YouTube and Flickr. If early cybercultural theory portrayed the body as absent within cyberspace, then Web 2.0 theory seems characterized by an emphasis on visibility. Today, the body's presence occupies the foreground through the visual display of the anorexic body via images, photographs, pictures and videos. Embodiment is reconstituted both narratively and visually via these new performances. Moreover, the anorexic body, which might otherwise be hidden, comes to be re-imagined in new ways:

> We don't know what a body is because a body is always in excess of our knowing it, and provides the ongoing possibility of thinking or otherwise knowing it. It is always in excess of any representation, and indeed, of all representations ... which doesn't mean that it is unthinkable but that we approach it in thought without fully grasping it.
>
> (Grosz 2001: 28)

While there is no 'corporeal immediacy' (Heim 1993), a physical presence cannot be simply bracketed off in these contexts, because these environments are virtual. For example, consider the following comments from one Pro-Ana member:

> [H]ello, does anyone want to share pics of their progress with me ... ? write me and let me know.
>
> (Anonymous user, Pro-Ana blog)

> [H]eres some pictures of me ... my hip bones have always stuck out alot even in my fat days.
>
> (Anonymous user, Pro-Ana blog)

Descriptions of the body in cyberspace like this one raise questions about the extent to which the body is definable (Kennedy 2000: 471). Drawing upon Virilio's work on new communication technologies, Mules (2000) suggests that the 'transmission of images takes place at such a rate that the past is collapsing into the present, creating an overpowering sense of immediacy'. Thus,

> we can no longer speak of the image as a representation ... rather, we need to think of the possibility of a kind of 'image-event' incorporating both the physical reality of the human body and its image, stretched through time and space.
>
> (ibid.)

From this perspective, the depiction of the anorexic body in cybermedical spaces cannot be considered to simply constitute some representation of it beyond virtual worlds. Rather, it takes on a presence within virtuality, as an 'image-event'. For example, in their ethnographic work on the Pro-Ana website Anagrrl, Fox *et al.* (2005b: 955) report that accompanying a photo of one user were captions about how the image might be 'disturbing' and 'crack the screen' because 'the participant was fat and undesirable'. Here, the virtual image takes on a 'being' in cyberspace beyond some signification or display. It takes on a presence that enacts a certain kind of physicality.

Approaching Pro-Ana in this way allows us to 'begin to ask questions about how the body is staged differently in different environments' (Balsamo 2000: 98). The anorexic body is particularly significant in terms of how we might understand a politics of cyberfeminism, and we return to these discussions in the remaining chapters of the text. Indeed, it leads us to theorize Pro-Ana and the medicalization of cyberspace more generally as a posthuman process, which is the focus of the next chapter. The anorexic body in cyberspace is not just a representation of the body but might also offer an ontological transformation of the anorexic body. Others (Ferreday 2003; Dias 2003; Fox *et al.* 2005a, b) have pointed out how photo-imagery in these spaces represents a method to make public the hidden anorexic body. In building on this perspective, our analysis above leads us to add that the anorexic body also takes on a new form and presence in cyberspace, which is 'no longer secondary to the thing it represented' (Mules 2000). In this sense, the re-imagining of the anorexic body and its new configuration in cyberspace emerges as a 'post-human manifestation' (Kennedy 2000: 15), constituted through new modes of subjectivity (Stryker 2000).

Contrary to theories that claim the body may disappear into text within cyberspace, many of the narratives constructed in these contexts offer alternative ways of *knowing* the body. In exploring these aspects of anorexia, we may better understand the active role that young women take in making sense of their subjectivities within and through anorexia (see Rich and Evans 2005). The emergence of these stories in an environment that is largely unregulated raises questions about the extent to which young women should be supported within wider health and education settings. For example, should spaces be available for young women with anorexia – and other disordered conditions of the body such as self-harm – to articulate these narratives? If so, is it also possible that this can or should be a regulated space, or must it emerge from active communities that fashion their own spaces of expression? Answering these questions becomes a matter of understanding what is 'unsayable and untellable in particular contexts' (Chase 1995: 24, cited in Dias 2003). While ethical discussion on these issues is embryonic, Pollack (2003: 250) takes the view that

> feminists who desire to address this issue may find it useful to engage with these women in their chosen community of cyberspace. ... Find ways in which we can use this medium to try to understand these women and with them collaboratively develop strong voices while maintaining healthy bodies.

Digital technologies not only present new modes of negotiation over the social construction of anorexia, but also provide a 'virtual laboratory for analysing the postmodern – and perhaps post-human – condition' (Robins 2000: 81). If we are to move beyond theories that pathologize and individualize eating disorders (Cogan 1999), then we need spaces within which we can hear things we may find uncomfortable, but which provide rich understandings of the complex processes of embodiment.[4] As Ferreday (2003: 288) argues, 'by attempting to build a community precisely through representing and speaking about minds and bodies that have been positioned as abject, Pro-Ana websites perform a model of community that explicitly refuses the project of becoming unmarked.' The body adopts a central role in these communities, not only through processes of monitoring, regulation, or modification (via the sharing of tips and tricks associated with anorexia), but also through the representation of the anorexic body in public spaces. In doing so, bodies that may usually remain hidden become visible and challenge the dichotomy between public and private. As Bury (2001: 274) notes, having spaces to express one's health narrative may be significant since it can often come to represent an '"ordering of experience" in the face of disruptive experiences' (Good 1994: 161). Thus, these spaces reveal a great deal about why young women seek support elsewhere.

9 The bioethics of cybermedicalization

Our posthumanist reading of Pro-Ana communities is a confrontation with bio-medical models of health, though it is necessary to elaborate on this reading more fully to explain our intentions in offering posthumanism as an analytical device. One of the central themes of our discussion on the medicalization of cyberspace has been an exploration of the relationship between ethical and social scientific analyses of medical or pseudo-medical practices that stretch the limits of medicine's traditional goals. While medicalization generally has been inscribed with sociological assumptions and developed in the context of cultural and social studies, it has clearly implied a concern that can be described as moral and ethical. Morally, the concern over medicalization involves the degree to which it limits the enjoyment of a fulfilling and enriched life, through its relegation of social problems to the surveillance of medical expertise. Ethically, there are concerns that the practice of medicine is stretching beyond its prescribed role and that this can diminish both the integrity of medicine and, ultimately, patient care.

In this chapter, we make this ethical context more explicit and offer explanations and responses to the positioning of ethics within medicalization work. To reiterate one of our earliest statements, we do not presume that medicalization is inherently negative or undermining of autonomy. We agree with Rose (2007: 700), who observes that 'since at least the 18th century in developed countries, medicine played a constitutive part in making up people'. Consequently, our ethical objection to it would be to object to the very conditions of existence that allowed the derivation of a medicalization discourse. Thus, Rose states that 'medicine has been fully engaged in making us the kinds of people we have become' and that 'this is not in itself grounds for critique'. We refer back to our earlier note on the comment of bioethicist Eric Juengst, who defines medicalization as *inherently* negative, since it is 'the mistake of applying the medical model to the wrong problem' (1998: 43). Our difficulty with this view is that there is considerable disagreement about whether a particular set of circumstances is, indeed, the wrong problem. So, if one were to talk about sexual dysfunction as a medicalized condition, the point of contention is often over whether a given set of circumstances is the effect of a treatable biological dysfunction rather than a social or psychological condition, for which the legitimacy of medical intervention is more dubious.

As was outlined in the previous chapter, anorexia and eating disorders more generally are often met with mixed responses to this matter. A range of conflicts of interest that are latent within the allied medical sciences and professions accompany these concerns. Thus, it is naïve to ignore the interest of pharmaceutical companies to support medicalization in so far as it leads to the utilization of their products. Also, one must take into account the interests of health care services to seek the most economical adequate solution to a given problem, given the limitation of resources. Finally, it is necessary to recognize that it is in the interest of patients to seek the least burdensome treatments. These factors strengthen the position of those who are concerned about medicalization, though the challenge seems to be more about how one discusses medicalization in the context of practices that might be described as lifestyle choices. To elaborate on this, it will be helpful to pursue more fully how one situates ethical concern in the context of Pro-Ana websites.

The ethics within Pro-Ana

Pollack's (2003: 249) recent work on what a feminist response to Pro-Ana might involve alludes to the dangers that 'postmodern feminists may romanticize these spaces as political statements and thus, in essence, condone the inherent self-destructiveness that such a protest entails'. She warns against 'the possibilities for the pro-anorexic subject becoming a symbolic martyr'. These concerns arise partly because the anorexic body enacts *the cyborg ritual* discussed earlier: 'a paradoxical situation in which the development of increasingly "natural" and embodied interfaces leads to "unnatural" adaptations or changes in the user' (Biocca 1997). Indeed, claims continue to be made that some Pro-Ana support groups have been found to foster rather negative competitions for weight loss (Chesley *et al.* 2003):

> [H]ow many of you thin hotties want to prove yourself ang gain personal satisfaction (not weight) by showing you are the best at getting rid of that shit that pull your self-steem even more down? well guess what? the best way of doing that is to compete!!! so lets do this, starting AUGUST 21 i am competing against anyone who will challenge me (friendly competition of course), for a chance to prova myself ... if you think you ca keep up, reply before the 21 and let me know ... this will help as motivation for you to lose more weight and reach your beloved numbers (lowest weight) so we will have fun!) we will be eating 500 or less calories ONLY IN FOOD THAT IS FRUIT OR VEGETABLE FOR THREE WEEKS STRAIGHT. the person who wins picks another competition. so if you are in, reply. ... YOU HAVE NOTHING TO LOSE IF YOU TRY TO COMPETE, ONLY POUNDS!!!!
>
> (Anonymous user, Pro-Ana blog)

Thus, the sort of ethical concerns about the Pro-Ana movement reflect a position that construes cyberspatial narratives not merely as discursive transformations,

but as sites that may prompt material and bodily change. Part of the critique lev-
elled at these communities is driven by concerns that they may foster competition
and secrecy among users. We would be cautious of drawing parallels between virtual communities and the observations that within real-time support groups,
members may negatively evaluate each other (see Walstrom 2000). Instead, we
emphasize the need for further online ethnographies of Pro-Ana and other health-
related communities.

Work on cybercommunities has already informed some of these discussions.
Numerous papers in this area discuss how social hierarchies of the body are established in computer mediated communication contexts, even without the presence
of actual visual body cues (see Wakeford 1999). Hierarchies connect with what is
valued and, in this sense, certain sets of meanings are created and sustained as
having value *across* the narratives of these young women, affording them not only
alternative subjectivities but relations of power and knowledge. As Mitra (1997:
59) suggests, 'Since the Internet user is empowered to play an active role in the
production of the discursive community, identity and community are formed
around the discourses that are shared by members.'

The juxtaposition of this potentially liberalizing movement with potentially
harmful implications is central to discussions concerning the gendered ethics of
medicalized cyberspace. These Pro-Ana cyberspaces challenge the medicalized
notions of anorexia, drawing upon embodied, gendered experiences. In particular,
they refute the traditional 'sick role whereby there is an obligation to seek and com-
ply with medical treatment, reducing the ill person to patient' (Frank 1997: 31).

In this sense, Pro-Ana may be a significant case for the development of cyberfeminist theory, since it occupies such a transgressive space (Dias 2003; Ferreday
2003). In part, this is also why we adopt a posthumanist reading of medicalized
cyberspace. The cases we outline provoke questions about how discursive practices and power over women's bodies and ill health are theorized. They draw
attention to the rewritings of, and on, the body, associated with particular subjectivities. However, the problem of the anorexic body, the Pro-Ana body, is that it
mediates liberal and radical feminisms in a way that might be negatively plural.
The idea of reconstituting one's subjectivity, of reconstituting the anorexic body
outside of psychiatric and biomedical discourse, is marred by the manner in
which such control is conducted and accepted. It is marred by the dangerous and,
perhaps, even life-threatening possibilities around body modification via self-
starvation. This is the basis on which these alternative narratives become rejected
as a legitimate discourse.

Fox *et al.* (2005b: 947) make a critical point in this discussion when noting that
Pro-Ana differs from other explanatory frameworks in rejecting the position that
anorexia is a wholly negative condition that must always be 'remedied through
medical treatments or psychosocial intervention'. Pro-Ana explicitly challenges
this and raises a critical question for the ethics of health care: should the recourse
to recovery be considered an absolute criterion by which we assess the expectations of these cyberspaces? Relativism may allow us to consider the biological
property rights of minority or subjugated groups, including the often silenced

voices of these young anorectics. These cyberspatial voices draw attention to the need for young women to have safe environments within which they can construct the often chaotic, embodied, and painful stories of anorexia. However, this should not imply a retreat to an epistemology of solipsism or absolute relativity on the ethics of anorexia. Drawing upon Braidotti (2002: 228), we do not wish to fall into either 'moral relativism [n]or the suspension of ethical judgement'.

To endorse the Pro-Ana position of supporting the rights of an individual to sustain anorexia at any stage of an eating disorder would be to support a position of extreme relativism characterized by a lack of shared understanding of treatment or prognosis and, perhaps, poststructural nihilism (Squires 1993). A position of absolute relativity, while supporting the Pro-Ana position, would preclude any shared understanding of how one should treat anorexia, if at all. Much like the Pro-Ana notion of *lifestyle choice,* rationality in this sense is determined by an individual's own experiences of the world. Conversely, as Pollack (2003: 249) suggests,

> a pedagogical solution of 'enlightening' these women about the oppressive nature of their embodied protest implicitly undermines their agency and thus perpetuates the current interplay of dominant cultural discourses that enticed the anorexic to take a pro-eating disorder stance in the first place.

Yet the contested terrain of this subject is about 'whether someone in the grip of an eating disorder can actually make competent decisions about their quality of life' (Draper 2000: 120). After all, Pro-Ana is a movement that embraces the idea that one can make competent decisions to live with anorexia and refuse treatment. However, as Draper (ibid.: 126) cautions, 'we should be wary of confusing irrational reasons with reasons with which we simply do not agree. Furthermore, we should be wary of confusing either irrationality or strong disagreement with incompetence'. Draper goes on to suggest that a biomedical model of health asserts that those with anorexia 'are not competent to make decisions that relate in any way to food and withdrawing therapy or treating palliatively effectively entails withdrawing feedings' (ibid.: 122). Certainly, there are legitimate moral and ethical reasons why medical intervention in the decisions that a young woman makes about her health is appropriate. But what of those individuals, like many of the cases outlined above, who are not 'broadly incompetent', who 'are studying for school leaving exams or degrees' (Draper 2000: 122) but choose to live their life in a state of starvation? Cyberspatial narratives highlight many of the complexities that mediate these discussions around ethics and the choice to engage in what are seen as problematic practices (such as self-starving). In large part, our medicalization of cyberspace is characterized by this phenomenon. By reading these narratives *alongside* wider cultural scripts about health and illness, they provide new cultural significations about the body and facilitate a dialectical relationship between the social and ethical. Exploring these narratives as alternative features of recovery is particularly important when we consider that despite massive study of and resources available for treating these potentially fatal conditions [eating disorders], they remain pervasive. ... The slow progress made in alleviating eating disorders becomes even more frightening, considering that these conditions are grossly underreported – both their occurrences and fatalities.

(Walstrom 2000: 762)

However, as Dias (2003) notes, most studies on recovery from eating disorders have been conducted within a biomedical model, exploring causes and treatments, focusing on the negative factors that might prevent recovery. She argues that what seems absent from the literature is a focus on positive outcome indicators, which are most likely to come in narrative form, rather than measurable indicators. Some authors are beginning to speculate on whether voicing one's desire to retain and embrace anorexia (as indicated in the Pro-Ana voices in Chapter 8) may be a productive aspect of the recovery process:

[A] statement that he [*sic:* the therapist] agrees that the patient is probably better off, all things considered, remaining anorexic, can be the most helpful and often totally new experience for the anorexic. She [*sic*] can approach the task of limited weight gain with much more confidence under such circumstances.

(Crisp, *anorexia nervosa, let me be,* cited in Draper 2000: 129)

These are uncomfortable and ethically complex circumstances to accept, requiring an unusual form of empathy with the experience of the sufferer.

Posthumanism: the absent present

These interpretations of the online Pro-Ana movement must be seen in the context of broader cybermedicalization issues. It is one example of how the virtualization of identity has led to a prostheticization of the body, which is revealed as a removal process towards an artificial prosthetic – a prosthetic that is designed to *not* fit, to be burdensome. This notion of a prosthetic burden returns us to the main theoretical premises of the book, where the medicalization of cyberspace encompasses the consideration of health outside of the traditional medical environment and within the multi-faceted, non-regulated (rather than unregulated) space of the Internet.

The medicalization of cyberspace embodies the way that medical practice is developing in the contested conditions of postmodernity, where ethical discourse takes place within a space of ambiguous realness. As Braidotti (2002: 2) observes, 'we live in permanent processes of transition, hybridization and nomadization, and these in-between states and stages defy the established modes of theoretical representation'. In keeping with these observations, we have not attempted to assert a single, comprehensive view of the body in cyberspace. Instead, we have explored how questions of materiality and humanness emerge via the context of medicalized cyberspaces. Through our examples, various modes of enacting what Sandberg (2001) describes as 'morphological freedom' have been articulated. The auctioning of a human kidney on eBay, the pro-anorexia movement and the rhetoric of the first human clone each clarify the broadening base of ethical concern and its challenge to social science.[1] This confrontation takes two forms, the first of which is most clearly espoused by Fuller's (2006) critique of 'bioliberalism,' as fundamentally antithetical to sociology's socialism. Fuller's concern is that the legitimization of such practices leads to a diminishing respect for human subjectivity, and his views are not unlike Fukuyama's (2002) attack on technoprogressive or transhumanist claims. Fuller's encounters with bioethics are part of a series of inquiries by social scientists who have become critical of the politics of bioethics. Over the past few years, a number of other sociologists have offered similar critiques of how bioethics should engage more fully with sociological issues (Haimes 2002; Hedgecoe 2004; de Vries *et al.* 2006; López 2004).[2]

The second confrontation involves the operable mode of sociology, as the study of societies. This is explained usefully through another example. In 2002, designers from the Royal College of Art in London developed a prototype of a telephone tooth implant that would sit permanently lodged in the tooth, rather like a cavity filling.[3] These designers had no intention of developing the product, and so in one sense the episode was a hoax (Metz 2006). Yet the media treated the concept as a genuine product that might arrive soon on the market. The imaginary artefact took on a life of its own and came to constitute the conditions within which such prospects came to matter to previously unengaged communities.[4] Indeed, with the increasing miniaturization of technology to the nano scale, the concept is difficult to dismiss outright, although such applications are nowhere near realization. Again, this reminds us of the examples discussed earlier in the context of David Cronenberg's film *The Fly* (1986). This provocation appeals to the kinds of blurred space that are now characteristic of discussions about the future, where technological possibility is treated as technological probability or inevitability.[5] Perhaps the height of the success for these designers was making the front cover of *Time* magazine, which confirmed the extent of their provocation.

Such future-casting advances the sociological criticisms of futurology in quite interesting ways, and these provocations are inextricable from an analysis of medicalized cyberspace.[6] Indeed, imagining the (ethical) future has become a more legitimate practice for sociologists via the recent trend towards upstream public engagement on science and technology issues, which has, in turn, provoked discussions about the value of *empirical ethics.*[7] While one might discuss the politics and sociology of these possible futures – bioliberalism versus bioconservativism – what seems uncontested is the rebiologization of sociology that the debate presumes. Indeed, Delanty (2002) takes stock of the challenge this provokes by considering how the science of genetics is inevitably socially constructed by individual agency, and so we must look to the social sciences to make sense of this. He goes on to locate these discussions in the context of a public discourse that resembles the upstream engagement debates about science.

Accompanying these conversations is the emerging conceptual lens of *mobility,* which Urry (2000) offers to explain how sociologists must work in a period that is characterized by the absence of societies. We will return to this concept in the conclusion, though it is useful to mention that an integral aspect of this work attends to the digital dimensions of mobile cultures. It offers further support for considering online health discourses as mechanisms through which to make sense of technological identity and its relationship to the officialdom of medicine. However, it is also important to link these ideas with other contemporary health care debates, such as the notion of *medical tourism,* where clients travel the world in search of medical laws that accommodate their particular need or desire. One can include our earlier discussions about body and organ trafficking within such debates.

Within cultural studies, there have been some precedents for these discussions about the ethics of bioliberalism, which we have already mentioned in various ways. Thus, conversations about cyborgs – more Kevin Warwick's enhanced human than Donna Haraway's interest in the differently able – have infused imaginative practices of cultural forecasting by aligning it with the established politics of cultural studies. For example, Gray appeals to the concept of the cyborg to address the interests of marginal groups whose humanness is not given full moral or legal recognition. His 'cyborg bill of rights' establishes that, among other things, there must be freedom of 'consciousness' and of 'family, sexuality, and gender' (2002: 28–29). His ideas and, more recently, Zylinska's (2005) relocation of ethics within cultural studies, culminating in her own manifesto for feminist cyberbioethics, stop short of utopian claims in order to argue on behalf of Otherness – of allowing people the freedom of biological modification in so far as it addresses plausible identity claims.

However, these manifestos are characteristic of an optimistic phase within the social sciences – the aspiration to study as yet unknowable societies.[8] In response to these discussions about the role of bioethics in social sciences (and vice versa), Zylinska's 'feminist cyberbioethics' retreats from what might be described as cyber-libertarianism or bioliberalism to a proposed study of the 'ethics of hybrids'. These ideas have clear connections with a range of literature, such as Butler's (1993) notion of 'bodies that matter' and Mary Douglas' (1965) thesis on 'matter out of place', whose work has been discussed recently in the context of biological modification (Coyle 2006). The Pro-Ana community also responds to this problematic, as it is constituted by the presence of medical knowledge out of its proper, regulated sphere and, arguably, beyond the reach of that sphere.[9]

Like Zylinska (2005), we also revert from the cyborg paradigm in order to apply a more precise, theoretical claim about the medicalization of cyberspace. This is because our claim is only partially connected to the cyborg metaphor (as *cyborg ritual*), which has become only one form of various ways of conceptualizing the implications of machinic interfaces with biology.[10] We also consider that Haraway's cyborg has often entered contemporary academic parlance without taking into account how non-central were her aspirations to talk about the imminence of the cyborg as a posthuman entity.[11] Rather, Haraway's ideal sits comfortably with the idea that there are fewer and fewer reasons to accept clarity over ontological distinctions.[12] Indeed, Haraway suggests as much when proclaiming that 'the cyborg is our ontology; it gives us our politics' (1991: 150), thus invoking our earlier claim about the presence of the anorexic body in Pro-Ana movements. In each of the cases we discuss, the cybernetic organism cannot be reduced to mere information; yet the body is both absent and present in cyberspace.

The concept of presence is a crucial, though contested, notion in studies of digital cultures. Stories of suicide chat rooms (Rajagopal 2004) suggest that communication about sensitive or private issues online can often be accompanied by a weak sense of responsibility in participants that works to counter the quality of the experience. This has implications for what we call the *bioethics of cybermedicine.* Discussions about physical presence are accompanied by criticisms of bioethics as an industry of sorts, which lacks a demonstrated ability to prioritize social needs – such as welfarist conceptions of health care (Purdy 2001; Turner 2003; Zylinska 2005).[13] To this, we also add the commercialization of ethical culture – shopping, eating, energy, tourism, etc. – as further evidence of how the ethical has become *hyphenated* in the sense offered by Žižek (2004), as a surrogate for *genuine* ethical concern. In this manner, the absent presence within bioethics is characterized by its overwhelming presence within the public sphere, and lacking any ability to argue on behalf of basic health care needs. We are both overwhelmed and unassisted by bioethics, to the point where key scholars in the midst of discussions about medicine's future are beginning to think 'beyond bioethics' (Fukuyama and Furger 2007). This situation also explains why our construction of the absent present is ethical: it is the presence of an ethical commitment within cultural studies, which is constituted by an absence of the capability to scrutinize judgements. This is not a criticism of pluralism as such, nor wholly a criticism of those who have pioneered bioethics. Indeed, it is more carefully an appeal to consider what literature should inform bioethical deliberations and to support Callahan (1993: S9) in his counsel that bioethics must continue to 'expand its own horizons'.[14]

Textual bodies

We have explored the complex interplay that occurs between embodied forms of subjectivity in cyberspace and have endeavoured to show how identities are medicalized through the Internet. We have offered various types of examples that achieve this. Some of our examples reveal how identities are medicalized through their reconfiguration of the relationship between old and new media and the expectations of each as truth makers and truth fakers. Other examples reveal a similar occurrence through their constituting counteractions to legitimate medicalizing phenomenon, as is suggested by the Pro-Ana communities, where self-help and community support are ambiguously read by expert discourses.

Theoretical notions of the textual human, which have been discussed in cyberspatial literature, are intimated by Hayles' (1999) suggestive notion of the posthuman, which privileges informational pattern over material instantiation. However, Hayles' notion may appear to misrepresent how medicalized identities are formed in cyberspace, particularly in relation to the cases of medicalization presented above. Cyberspace is an environment impoverished of flesh and, yet, it is a space within which there is a continual engagement with body matters, including health, reproduction, body disorder, and so on. In this sense, cyberspace is the body reincarnate, with essential missing or transformative ingredients. As processes of medicalization operate in cyberspace, one is drawn into a perpetual engagement with body matters, though in an environment where the body is sometimes considered to be missing. As such, these processes invoke and embody an ongoing sentimental search for bodily attributes. As Kroker and Weinstein (1994) describe,

> Why be nostalgic? The old body type was always OK, but the wired body with its micro-flesh, multi-media channeled ports, cybernetic fingers, and bubbling neuro-brain finely interfaced to the 'standard operating system' of the Internet is infinitely better. Not really the wired body of sci-fi with its mutant designer look, or body flesh with its ghostly reminders of nineteenth-century philosophy, but the hyper-texted body as both: a wired nervous system embedded in living (dedicated) flesh.

Prosthetic burdens

Our analysis claims that the body is neither obsolete, as Stelarc (1997) proclaims, nor does it 'no longer exist' (Kroker and Kroker 1987); the digital form does not obscure the body. Instead, it enables the development of an alternativee, *prosthetic* body to emerge, which brings with it both new and old burdens. As Braidotti (2002: 227) notes, 'today's body is immersed in a set of technologically mediated practices of prosthetic extension'. However, before we explain this further, it is necessary to clarify the meaning of prosthesis and why we claim that a new form of prosthetic – to replace the last prosthesis, Viagra – is a useful articulation of cyberspace's medicalization, compared with cyborg manifestos.

Prostheses are artificial devices that replace absent (body) parts, though virtual bodies lack no visual parts. The 'missing part' is imag(in)ary, again, and the (ab)users pursue some truth of being that is entirely fabricated. The sites of these medicalized, prosthetic identities are hypothetical cyberspace communities. Notably, however, the Web does *not* play a constructive role here. Rather, the underlying ideologies embodied by cyberspaces reflect the mediatory nature of cyberspace. The images are indicative of a broader synthetic that is valued because it defies its designation as *virtual,* as non-reality. This is the discourse that drives Hayles' (1999) informational human. The cyberspatial prosthetic is an informational prosthetic, necessarily a mask for some*one* rather than some*thing.*

In this sense, the body-self narratives of young anorectics operate within a 'mediated co-presence, where the real and the virtual enmesh and interact' (Mules 2000). Thus, our language for engaging the cybermedical problematic resists the complete overcoming of cyborgisms in favour of an emerging prosthetic, outlined in various recent texts (see Smith and Morra 2006). We do not advance the idea that online discussion boards or blogs are indicative of bodies becoming less *fleshy,* or neutralized into mere information. Rather, we articulate them as ambiguously transformative, absent but present. As Wright (1999: 24) indicates, '"I" may become text, seemingly free of gender or racial identity, but both text and fluid identity remain prosthetic'. Extending Wright (1999: 23), we have argued that the cybermedicalization of the body is a further 'step towards the de-politicisation of gender'. In this sense, it can be characterized as *post*-gender, but not *past*-gender. It is a critical reworking of gender boundaries, rather than the complete effacing of them. It also provides a reason for scepticism over the distinctiveness of cyberfeminism as a discrete discourse. To reiterate our earlier point, prostheticization does not lead to the effacing of gendered discourses, but is the means through which to rework some of the boundaries.

Conclusion

After-cyborgs or artificial life

Itinerant healers are returning. They will ride the information superhighway.
(Mitchell 1995: 75)

This work began in 2002 and emerged out of a concern that institutions and professions were reacting to the Internet in a defensive – and subsequently offended – mode. These reactions seemed to contradict what ought to be the explicit commitments of such institutions. Yet they also conveyed one of the central problems with the Internet's contribution to society, which is its confrontation to the non-virtual knowledge hierarchies that are fashioned through systems of expertise, authority, professionalization and institutionalization. Within the cultural study of health and medicine, as further studies of medicalization were emerging, the Internet seemed to be one critical context that had been omitted from the analysis. Yet an increasing colonization of the Internet by the professions was already taking place.

At the conclusion of this book, we signal our interest in conveying new directions for theoretical work on digital culture, in the context of the sociology of health and posthumanism. We have discussed a range of cybermedical phenomena, which are similar in their having occupied spaces of ambiguously or partially regulated medical spectacle. Our aim was to theorize and document these emerging cultures of cybermedicalization and to understand what happens when they clash with the regulatory aspirations of the allied health professions. We have suggested a theoretical foundation to cybermedical sociology that takes into account ideas within studies of medicalization, digital culture, bodies and technology, and the role of ethics within these debates. However, there is a considerable amount of literature that we have omitted from our analysis, which is broadly reflected in the excellent work of the *Journal of Medical Internet Research* (*JMIR*). Here, authors undertake research into the utility of digital systems to deliver health care and the challenges this raises. Moreover, they provide empirical evidence that informs our understanding of the extent and manner of cybermedical utilization. In places, the evidence within this journal supports our claims, while other studies reveal the limited use of digital systems across some demographics. Yet in all cases the complexity of conceptualizing cybermedicine is evident, as are the continuing concerns about reliability, trustworthiness and inclusion/exclusion.

In contrast to this work, we have developed an understanding of the trend towards cybermedicalization, a project the relevance of which is borne out by the existence of *JMIR*. Of considerable significance to us has been the range of technophobia that accompanies cybermedical events. We have worked towards a conceptual framework that takes into account the limitations of claims that such events are indicative of a *past*-human era, and yet we have attempted to acknowledge the embeddedness of digital worlds within the non-digital. There is, we argue, less value in arguing on behalf of a separation of these two characteristics but, importantly, this does not mean that we are all *hard* cyborgs. Indeed, we share the concerns expressed by Sundén (2001: 216), who indicates a frustration over claims that theoretical perspectives on new technologies imply the transformation of everyday lives:

> How can discursive transformations in narratives ... lead to material transformations and social change? Asking these questions is not to undervalue theoretical work, or the way we live by fictions, in the name of some more 'real' and solid material reality. Rather it is a way to show that there might be a weak link between the feminist cyborg and the reality where women who use the new technology find themselves. For what happens to political action when the only politics in sight are deeply anchored in the story of the cyborg body?

Instead, we argue on behalf of *post*-humanism, which expresses a critical stance towards the polarization of views on the ethics of emergent technological cultures. Our cases speak to specific instances of this posthumanism, though they are by no means exhaustive. To this extent, it might be mistaken to speak about *cultures* of cybermedicalization, since we have not developed a typology of communities and practices. Nevertheless, there exist medicalized cyberspaces that are characterized by the notion of becoming; they involve a process of negotiation on body and health issues where 'online bodies are bodies that are certainly being written, but simultaneously bodies to write on' (Sundén 2001: 229). In the stories we describe, women are no longer merely the 'machine parts' (ibid.: 219) of the human–computer interface, but are made 'more autonomous' (ibid.) through their 'symbiotic relationship to machines' (ibid.).

We have studied forms of medical space that have invaded cyberspaces and we have exposed the consequences of this blurring of boundaries. Our debates have centred on crucial discussions within socio-political studies of the Internet, which emphasize difficulties surrounding the definition and regulation of public and private space – such as the notion of expertise, authority and authenticity. The Internet, as a doctor's surgery or hospital, becomes an interesting metaphorical lens through which to conceptualize the range of contexts that pervade medicalized cyberspace. However, this conceptualization invokes an expectant regulative framework that is not necessarily sensible to apply.

Beyond this clash of counter-cultures, theoretical work on medicalized cyberspace must draw on a range of issues that derive from or are derivative of debates surrounding the technological body: the cyborg, transhuman and posthuman. We have not been particularly concerned with theorizing these different, but related, concepts, which is done elsewhere (Miah 2008). However, we have discussed the tendency of online spaces to be framed by these concepts in their varied guises. This is situated in the ambivalence expressed within contemporary culture and cultural practices towards technology. The revealing of the cybercultures we have described prompts fears of automation, in so far as it indicates the effacing of human dignity and a general technological overcoming of humanity. Yet the participants within these cybercultures do not observe the technological systems that they are using as unwelcome, or antithetical to their biological identity. Rather, this is the character given to cybercultures via their constitution as forms of media spectacle. The stories are authenticated, first, by their being located within the Otherness of cyberspace and, second, in the unfamiliar terrain of the technology itself.

For the user, the technological space forms part of their lifeworld, perhaps in the same way that mobile phone technology extends the body's communicative capacity. Indeed, increased mobility is a crucial justification for further studies into cybermedicalization, and various examples already suggest how mobility will be a crucial characteristic of emerging health care practices. As was noted earlier, Urry's (2000) characterization of mobile societies closely resembles the fluidity of our cybermedicalized narratives. Indeed, this process of naturalizing cyberspace technology can also be described in biological terms. For example, the technological character of cybermedicine is naturalized, rather like blood during a *transfusion*. The systems of communication become the *form* and the *mode* of our experience, and when this occurs we are all too human – we are posthuman – and indifferent towards the impositions of technology.

This leads us to explain the title for our conclusion, as an exploration of more suitable concepts through which to conceptualize the posthuman paradigm. Intimations of such a language come from the study of Artificial Life (AL), the paradigmatic theoretical model for future cybernetic systems and their integration with quotidian computer platforms (Helmreich 2001). The connections between digital technologies and broader biomedical spheres are visible in a number of cultural and artistic endeavours. For instance, Stelarc's *Prosthetic Head* relies on artificial intelligence to enable a surrogate conversation with the artist, albeit via a three-dimensional graphical rendering of his head. In support of this digital paradigm, Graham (1999: 420–421) notes that

> [t]he ubiquity of computer technology and electronic media and the advent of genetic engineering are extending and displacing the physical body into new media such as cyberspace, and reconfiguring taken-for-granted patterns of physical space, procreation, communication and intimacy.

The philosophy of Artificial Life involves a rejection of the traditional artificial intelligence (AI) model for building new life-entities, along with its ideological presumptions. In contrast, its bottom-up principles aim to *evolve* complexity by mimicking nature, rather than by imposing a model of the natural upon a machinic system. AL is after-cyborgs also, because it is theoretically progressive;

not a *hard* cyborg, but a life infused with (imperceptible) technology. Steadily, digital systems have become ubiquitous, though we frequently fail to perceive these systems as technology. AL is also a non-masculinist paradigm, where architects are busy building 'companion species' (Haraway 2006a), rather than better humans.

The medical professions and governments alone cannot respond to the consequences of further medical encounters online. Indeed, neither should there be an expectation for them to monitor such environments, which more closely resemble the communicative space of private or public conversations, rather than formal medical arenas. As Furedi (2004: 415) indicates, there is cause to be sceptical of the trend towards requiring professional involvement in matters of 'pain, disappointment and difficult transitions'. However, the professions should be concerned about becoming excluded (deliberately or otherwise) from these discussions, as this can imply some degree of mistrust over the medicalization of cyberspace. In this context, our stories require a retheorizing of the role of practices of medicine and medical technology in society.

There are many other aspects of medicalized cyberspace that require further consideration. For instance, over the past few years a closer relationship between the computer games industry and medical imaging solutions has emerged. In part, this has translated into greater legitimacy for the former, by suggesting the positive effects of game playing, but also via their wider connection to the virtual society. It has also reinforced the idea that interaction with technological systems can only be advanced through creative, collaborative solutions. The debates surrounding Web 2.0 are further indications of this, as emerging websites more effectively constitute the democratization of technology that the Internet promises. However, it is also important to recognize that the same trends of new media corporations continue to occur, thus placing limits on the claim that new media are separate from old. It is also important to recognize that many platforms that promise such freedom are also capable of 'mashing' a considerable amount of private data that could be used in ways that users do not realize. Alternatively, while we have mentioned mobile technologies to some extent, the prospects for transforming the delivery of health care have hardly been addressed. In part, this is because many of these prospects are not yet realized. We do not yet have structures that enable patients to interact with their doctors using 3G, though one can envisage that this will transform the meanings one ascribes to cybermedicine. Already, video sites such as Dr Pod are offering medical guidance via podcasting that will reach the prospective patient directly.

Finally, Part I indicated that our thesis operates at the precipice of a range of lifestyle modifications that can also be described as human enhancements. Considerably more work is inevitable in considering how such modifications connect with our medicalized cyberspaces and, indeed, with our cases. For instance, developments in nanotechnology suggest ways of altering eating patterns that could give rise to the application of such treatments for patients with anorexia. Nevertheless, our emphasis has been to discuss the cultures of computing that precede biomedicalization. In so doing, we have sought to foreground the era of biomedicalization through our discussion of examples such as Viagra and the auctioning of body parts. We indicate that this next stage of cybermedicalization has already begun to occur through the development of digital implants and nano devices. However, a more extensive consideration of this form of cybermedicalization will be the subject of another book, once these technologies make their way into our everyday world.

Afterword

Emma Rich

I would like to conclude our manuscript with a more personal narrative about the emerging relationship between health, illness and cyberspace. In 2003, my father died of a rare form of cancer called mesothelioma. Throughout my father's illness, the Internet played a central role in how my family made sense of and experienced his condition. Over these months, we found ourselves using the Internet to search for advice and information. We also joined support groups, which eventually served as a resource for coping with bereavement and mobilizing awareness of this particularly rare form of cancer. It is this narrative, albeit brief, I wish to offer as an afterword to our text, in order to make public an illness story that, like many stories of ill health, death and disease, would otherwise go untold. It speaks to many issues, not least of which is how processes of cybermedicalization impact upon patients' and carers' understandings of illness within the context of particular social relationships and medical structures.

Mesothelioma is a rare cancer affecting mesothelial cells, which cover the outer surface of most of the internal body organs, forming a lining that is sometimes called the mesothelium. Mesothelioma is caused by the inhalation of asbestos fibres. A short exposure can be enough, and the disease may lie dormant for up to forty years before symptoms begin to show. My father had worked for most of his adult life on building sites, and contracted mesothelioma through exposure to asbestos fibres within these environments. He died only three months after the initial diagnosis of his illness.

For around a year prior to his diagnosis, my father experienced various but continued symptoms of ill health and made regular visits to his local doctor. For months, he was lacking energy, suffering from chest infections and coughs, struggling to breathe, and experiencing weight loss and sleepless nights. Frequent prescriptions seemed to be masking what my father described as 'something more sinister' – this being what we later found out to be his own metaphor for terminal illness. He approached his doctor's appointments with both expectation and trepidation that he would eventually have some explanation for his persistent flu-like symptoms, and talked of needing some diagnosis to counter fears he would be seen as a hypochondriac. During this time, he had become increasingly frustrated that the medical community were not 'hearing him'. He wanted not only medical diagnosis, but to be included in the negotiation over the state of his own body, for health experts to hear his stories of pain, confusion, discomfort, and distress, and the intrusion and disruption that his illness was having on his everyday life and on people who cared for him. Initially, he felt that many of his concerns were being dismissed, signed away with another prescription. On other occasions, he came away from his appointments satisfied that doctors had been more responsive, the interaction involved less medical dominance, and that the experts were responsive and listened to his concerns and experiences.

As his condition worsened and we all became increasingly frustrated by our lack of understanding, my family decided to spend some time searching on the Internet for possible conditions related to his symptoms. As we optimistically stepped into a medicalized cyberspace, our search engine returned endless pages of online doctors, informational websites and self-diagnosis tools, all infused with technical medical language describing an array of possible illnesses and conditions.

Around the same time, my father's doctor had referred him to the hospital for a series of tests and scans. Not long after this, we all gathered in the specialist's office to be given the results of these procedures. In this brief meeting, we were informed that the results had revealed that he had mesothelioma, and given a very brief account of how this might have developed; this conversation was concluded quickly with the statement that this illness was currently incurable. I recall how not only my father as a patient, but all of us, invested significance in every gesture, pause, intonation of the specialist as she passed on her diagnosis. There was little she could tell us; no certainty or explanation about how long he might have left to live, what could be done to treat his condition, so we found ourselves scrambling for additional meaning in expression. This interaction was, no doubt, one of the many that this specialist would undertake in the course of her everyday duties in the medical profession, but it involved a series of what Komesaroff (1995: 69) refers to as microethical decisions about diagnosis: the kind of information given to my father as patient, and the manner in which it was expressed; the way in which our participation in the decision-making process was obtained and the specialist's engagement with us in relation to our views, questions, and so on. The specialist gave us minimal information in terms of what might be expected in relation to pain, discomfort, time, or ways to ease the patient, and us, through this illness.

After a cursory discussion about expected quality of life and treatment, my family pressed even further about what could be done. We were, unconvincingly, told of developments in science and technology and of emerging clinical trials, and given the restitution narrative that typically accompanies a diagnosis of cancer. We listened to the usual stories of strength, of beating the disease, and how there were cases where patients had continued to live well beyond what was expected. This felt more like a moral imperative to 'rise to the occasion' (Frank 1997) than any substance for hope. We were told of these stories perhaps not so much to express the success rate of those who survive mesothelioma, but more as part of the cultural expectation that one should encourage someone facing terminal illness to be complicit to a will to want to 'fight or beat the C word'. The delivery of this diagnosis was a critical moment and a memory for all of us, one that we revisited throughout the course of taking care of my father. It left a lasting impression on our understanding of the medical profession, the illness and each other. This was not simply a medical diagnosis, or the transmission of information; it set firmly in place our understanding of the cancer, our relationship with each other, our initial approach to managing it and, perhaps most significantly, a moment of major disruption to my father's sense of self. It involved the relinquishing of a certain self, the self that felt ultimately autonomous and in control of his health.

My father repeatedly tried to resolve the 'injustice' that he felt upon hearing this news, after a life in which he had accepted the moral duty of taking care of his health, eating well, not smoking, staying active, to be now faced with terminal illness. He referred back to this interaction during the times we talked about his cancer, recalling this moment as both an awakening, and on occasion of disruption and perplexity. It was this perplexity and uncertainty that propelled us to search for more information about mesothelioma. 'Perhaps if we ourselves go in search of more information' became our usual comforting narrative of hope – and so we found ourselves frequently online in this quest. Family members searched for every grain of knowledge, entering unsuspecting key words in search engines. Many of the search results produced further questions, but also supplied tools to help in terms of understanding this unusual condition, but also in having a supportive network of family and friends of other sufferers.

Initially, we visited what we might describe as medicalized sites, which described in technical medical discourse the condition, its aetiology, and clinical treatments. As we broadened our searches, we found ourselves shifting our collection of information away from the exclusive domain of the medical profession, towards personal embodied accounts of people experiencing this illness. We explored websites and discussion forums created by patients, and carers of those with mesothelioma. We read narratives about success stories, and more alarming stories that gave us a sense of the disordered, painful moments that might be endured. These stories tended to act as a form of 'informational medicine' whereby patients can become *producers* of health knowledge (Nettleton 2004). We found ourselves accessing information that, perhaps, would have been otherwise unavailable via the medical profession.

The more we read these accounts, as we visited websites, discussion forums and support groups, the more we seemed to make sense of these experiences in an ambiguous state. On the one hand, we invested a great deal in the medical domain, hoping it would provide comfort, answers and perhaps even some miracle treatment. Indeed, as my father's body began to break down and he was no longer able to care for himself, the ostensibly undeniable effectiveness and dominance of the medical domain, its knowledge, machinery, technology, became even more significant. It took on new meaning, and became literally embodied: drips that feed, specialists who decide and determine, drugs that ease. This was body and machine meeting, but through an integration of technology, science and illness.

But in its failure to offer solutions, answers or comforting knowledge, my family also found that science health care and objectivity were now thinly veiled. We found ourselves making sense of this illness and the experiences via different forms of health knowledge – from the technical, formal and objective 'medical' knowledge, to the embodied, disordered, painful but more humanistic stories of other sufferers.

In hindsight, it is difficult not to question which frameworks of knowledge become empowering, damaging, etc. in different moments and contexts. I often left the hospital or the computer terminal wondering whether diagnosis, labelling, knowledge and the medicalization of his illness were helpful or not. Diagnosis brought medicalization, but also a particular social understanding of the illness and treatment options. It seemed that, with my father, the diagnosis was disabling. Once he had been told of the severity of his sickness, he was haunted by this; it led to a sense of hopelessness. It seemed only to feed some unbroken continuum of despair and distress. Even now, I am unsure whether his awareness contributed in some way to such a rapid decline in his health. On one visit, it seemed that my father was confused by his condition and unaware of the severity of his illness. It seemed it had not been fully explained to him in this instance. On this visit, he was tearful, confused and in pain. It seemed that the specialist had made a decision about what would be in the best interests of him, as a patient. Just as the doctor faced these sorts of microethical decisions, we were also faced with choices regarding the knowledge we were acquiring via cyberspace. Would the knowledge of others who were in a more painful, serious and critical condition have added anything positive to his making sense of how to manage and prepare for his deteriorating body? On the one hand, the narratives we found on the Internet offered an explanation to make sense of the suffering body, of how we might approach it, address and treat it. But with this knowledge came a series of microethical choices we would have to make: Would we pass on this information? Would this not compound the social and personal distress, the fear of what would happen, of the degenerative body, grief? Would he want to hear of the uncertainties that exist in this field, how unpleasant an experience treatment itself might be, how pain, morbid fears and anxieties, and the disordered body intersect in ways that are often unfamiliar to us as patient, caregiver to significant other, the loss of dignity and privacy? Likewise, we could have selectively passed on hopeful stories of success, of the people who were living seven years on since their diagnosis of mesothelioma.

Many questions were raised at these junctures: would hearing success stories just place more of a moral imperative on my father to try to 'live successfully ill' and 'rise above' the dreaded C word, when what he needed was to express the despair he felt? Would this have impacted on his feeling that he could not construct an alternative narrative because of the fear, shame and guilt of not wanting to 'fight or beat the illness'? These were all microethical decisions that my family had to make, that typically accompanied the penetration of new forms of knowledge that were readily available to us through cyberspace. Our use of the Internet to make sense of this condition was embodied; not only was it contingent upon the very specific needs of having mesothelioma, but also it directly impacted upon the ways we approached aspects of care. Our considerations about passing on information we acquired were deliberated in relation to the reassurance they might offer, of the emotional impact as well as their more technical and pragmatic implications.

After my father's death in November 2003, the Internet still provided an important network and, perhaps, even a medium through which members of my family could express grief and bereavement. Our worlds had been irrevocably changed by this experience, not only through loss, but also through our understanding of bodies, medicine, health, illness, frailty, the delicate nature of deterioration.

Notes

Preface

1 We avoid any problematic assertion as to whether this change was the Internet's second, third or fourth change, and our use of the term 'Web 2.0' makes no intended claim either. Rather, we utilize it in recognition of how it has become used as a way of characterizing a number of emerging platforms that are achieving new opportunities for developers and users.

2 RSS involves Web feed formats that publish frequently updated content such as blog entries, news headlines or podcasts. This content may be published as either a summary or full text, and provides the user with automated updates.

3 This refers to the phenomenon of attempting to achieve a US size zero in women's clothing. This term was also associated with the fashion industry and received growing public attention following the Madrid Fashion Week in 2006, when models with a body mass index below 18 were prohibited from taking part in the event.

4 We use the concept of medical identity to refer to those aspects of identity that concern the knowledge and experience of wellness and sickness, which incorporates knowledge about conditions that are far removed from oneself.

Introduction: Medicine *in* society

1 It is useful to note the facility offered by computer-generated imagery in representing prehistoric life. Such films as *Jurassic Park* and subsequent documentaries draw on a similar narrative about the unknown may be constructed via technological imagination.

2 Like Woodward (1999: 282), we consider the discourse on losing control to be neglectful of how technology is 'embedded in social processes'.

3 This is not to reduce Google to information, but merely to explain how search engines differ in principle from journalism or, more specifically, journalists.

4 The complexity of the divide is grounded by Nettleton *et al.* (2004), who develop a 'typology' of users.

5 For instance, we consider using a telephone's Web browser to find an address or telephone number to be quite shallow use. In contrast, using the same device to connect with an online community through a chat facility is some measure of embeddedness within an online environment.

6 Given that this book is about medicine and the Internet, it would be interesting to discuss the relative importance of access to either 'information' or 'health services', though perhaps the common moral implication of each of these concepts is a further rationale for considering how they are related.

7 Of course, this positioning becomes increasingly problematic as the mass media (talk radio and reality TV) immerses itself further into online cultures.

1 Medicalization *in* cyberspace

1 We introduce the word 'unwanted' here to take into account Garry's (2001) observations on developing a critical account of medicalization that does not necessarily imply a rejection of medicine or even medicalized decision making. Thus, it is possible to accept aspects of medicalization while remaining generally critical of its process and its tendency to give rise to unwanted medical interpretations to social circumstances.

2 Nevertheless, since we are interested in the interface between cultural theory and bioethics, we note that the bioethics scholar Juengst (1998: 43) refers to medicalization as an inherently negative concept: 'the mistake of applying the medical model to the wrong problem'.

2 The cyborg body

1 We do not present this as support for Barlow's claim, but to reinforce this systematic construction of expectations about the Internet.

2 We might describe this as a 'sociology of the future' of which some Web studies became a part.

3 We are cautious about using this term, since it has become increasingly defunct as part of the language to describe personal websites. In anticipation that it will have no currency to some readers, homepages were simply personal websites. They occupy the same conceptual ground as something like Facebook or a MySpace account, though homepages were generally created, designed and maintained by individuals who had either self-trained in html or were beginning to use the WYSIWYG (What You See is What You Get) platforms, such as Microsoft's Frontpage or Macromedia's Dreamweaver. For a detailed study of how imagining audiences makes Web design a meaningful practice, see Hine (2001).

4 It is not untypical to engage non-cyberspecialists in debate about the Internet, whereby the conversations gravitate towards whether the Internet changes everything or nothing.

5 Indeed, this was a central component of the debate over whether its broadcaster, Channel 4, was culpable of producing racist content. If the programme is categorized as light entertainment, then the claim might stand. However, if it is evaluated as factual entertainment, then a different set of expectations and standards might apply.

6 We anticipate the claim that daily newspapers and even televised news coverage have an ephemeral quality from the perspective of the viewer or reader. Nevertheless, we are writing about publishing from the perspective of authors who endeavour to reach audiences, rather than viewers or readers who aim to access information. In this sense, their similarities are diminished.

7 We do not believe that the owners of such intellectual property (IP) encounter any loss as a result of this. Indeed, one might claim that their IP is enhanced by this brief, but high impact visibility.

8 In itself, this raises interesting opportunities for bringing together a range of methodologies and disciplines. For instance, the practice-based research debates within the United Kingdom have been particularly concerned with media productions, documentary, and so on. Mobile communication devices raise new questions about the distinction between theoretical and practical media studies, since image- and video-based data are becoming a core part of new media studies.

9 The subject of our analysis should not be that the teleportation went wrong, but that DNA of different species was mixed.

10 For examples, recent statements by Ulrich Beck and Donna Haraway each indicate the frustration with the new.

11 For more analysis of the Visible Man as criminal, see Cartwright (1997: 129), who discusses his 'public exoneration through his service-in-death to medical science and to public health culture'.

3 Cybermedicine and reliability discourse

1 A comparable analytical claim is found in Wyatt *et al.*'s (2005) use of Bakardjieva's notion of the 'warm expert' – 'someone with technical competence who is in a position to help a new internet user. A warm expert mediates between the specialized knowledge and skills necessary to use the technology and the specific situation and needs of the "novice" with whom the warm "expert" has some kind of more personal relationship' (Wyatt *et al.* 2005: 204).
2 Kedar *et al.* (2003: 326) suggest that 'Internet based consultations between specialists at centres of excellence and referring doctors contribute to patient care through recommendations for new treatment and timely access to specialist knowledge'.
3 This is also visible in Smith and Manna (2004).
4 For example, Hardey (1999) reports the case of one website called Quackwatch: 'Constructed by a retired psychiatrist and other sympathetic doctors in the United States the mission of Quackwatch is to warn users about what is regarded as unscientific or inappropriate health information. The site rejects all but "proven" medical material following a review by clinicians, and includes examples of unsound health material. ... Over a hundred dubious practices are listed and include acupuncture and traditional Chinese medicine' (Hardey 1999: 829–830).

4 Virtual governance of health behaviour

1 As others have noted, simply stated, 'obesity' refers to an excess of body fat and is to be distinguished from 'overweight', which refers to weight in excess of some standard. Brownell (1995: 386) emphasizes, 'measuring weight is easy and inexpensive, while measuring body fat is not.'
2 Body mass index is a tool used to measure and determine levels of obesity. A BMI score is calculated by weight in kilograms divided by height in metres squared (World Health Organization 1998). The index score is then used to determine an individual's weight (and health) category against the highly questionable concept of 'ideal weight': 'the idea that weight associated with optimum health and longevity could be determined by height' (Seid 1994: 7). BMI is now widely acknowledged to be imprecise, for example, it overestimates fatness in people who are muscular or athletic, it is not a good index for children and adolescents, it takes no account of age, sex or ethnicity, nor does it measure the levels of fat of an individual (see Evans *et al.* 2003b; Monaghan 2005). Despite this, it continues to be widely accepted and used as a measuring device because it is far easier to measure 'weight' than to measure 'fat', so BMI can be calculated quickly by the lay public without the use of expensive equipment.
3 These health discourses invoke the notion of 'agentic', which connects the healthy citizen with a particular and problematic version of selfhood. As Martin (2004: 200) suggests: 'Instead of an historically and socio-culturally situated concern for self-governance within a collective, morally and politically contested life world, we are offered a much more generic and apparently straight forward conception of self-management that seems largely within the control of individuals with the proper psychological attitudes and strategies'. In this sense, a type of humanist agency is invoked, which suggests that individuals are capable of detached masterful control in relation to health behaviour.
4 See http://news-service.stanford.edu/news/1998/june17/medsports617.html, *Journal of the American Medical Association*, 10 June 1998. The form was developed in 1997 by Dr Julie Peltz, a clinical fellow in sports medicine and postdoctoral fellow at the Stanford Center for Research in Disease Prevention. Peltz emphasized that a key goal in developing the form 'was not just to screen for participation risks such as sudden cardiac death but to provide a more comprehensive health assessment for adolescents'.

5 Cyberpatients, illness narratives and medicalization

1 Other conditions include '[e]ndometriosis, premenstrual syndrome, vaginal infections, uterine prolapse, cervical and endometrial cancer and problems of menopause' (Broom 2001: 256).
2 Similarly, Weisgerber (2004) explores how members of an electronic bulletin board devoted to sleep paralysis use the Internet to construct the phenomenon of sleep paralysis, and thereby contribute to a cultural agreement concerning what sleep paralysis is.

6 Partial prostitution

1 We draw on Zylinska (2005) in making this claim, whose ideas are explored later in the book.
2 A more substantive claim is made by a range of artists who employ prosthetics as a critical part of their pursuit – for example, the Catalan artist Neil Harbisson, whose prosthetic device is included within his passport photograph as confirmation of its permanent and embedded cyborg status. It seems important also to mention Laurie Anderson as a precursor to Harbisson's interaction with the aesthetics of music. Indeed, Anderson's recent experience as NASA's first artist in residence offers a range of connections with our discussions about expertise in matters of science, technology and medicine.
3 For a more detailed analysis of this component of eBay, see Robinson and Halle (2002). The authors also spend time detailing a case of a bogus painting that was auctioned on eBay, which raises parallel issues to the present inquiry.
4 For others since then, see Caplan (2004).
5 Turney (1998: 211) notes that claims about the first human clone appeared in 1978, also as an attempt to provoke public discussion. Also, Callahan (1998) indicates that discussions about the prospect also surfaced in the 1960s, after the cloning of the salamander. He notes that, at this time, the renowned co-discoverer of DNA James Watson speculated on the possible extension of cloning to humans.
6 This is not the case when looking at the same website today, which comes across as considerably outdated in design terms and, for this reason, suspicious.
7 Indeed, one might claim that the traditional media are ambushed by new media, and this reveals something about the inadequacy of journalistic practice and its tendency to interpret social significance into stories.

7 Biological property rights in cyberspace

1 Some of these issues are explained most successfully in the Russian film, *4*, directed by Ilya Khrjanovsky (2005) and written by renowned playwright Vladimir Sorokin. The film engages with cloning, though successfully operates outside of popular science fiction tropes to consider the interface of technological utopia *with* a concurrent dystopia. In this film, the authenticity of being human, unique, different, old, new, traditional, modern and the complicity of consumerism confront aspects of intense social control, as cloning is explained within a complex, imprecise and still mundane society.
2 Notably, Conrad (2005) emphasizes that medicalization should not be attributed to merely the medical professions, but also the commercial industries on which they depend.
3 Incidentally, Croissant (2006) notes that the product was developed to treat chest pain (angina) and that its utility for erectile dysfunction was accidental.
4 However, it is also important to recognize the lack of regulation of other controlled substances and products, such as tobacco (Banthin *et al.* 2004), and to take into account the possibility that the Web is a particularly appealing mechanism through which to advertise such products (Hong and Cody 2002).

5 We consider this to apply more generally to the shift from medical therapy to enhancement – a further expansion of medical liberties. The concerns about this are raised by
Fukuyama (2002).
6 As Hayles describes, the body is 'the original prosthesis we all learn to manipulate'
(1999: 3).

8 The online Pro-Ana movement

1 Dias (2003) suggests that some of these more moderate websites may not actively
encourage visitors to develop or maintain anorexia, but may focus more generally on
how to safely maintain anorexia, and offer support to those experiencing it. These
other sites take the position that some sufferers may be willing, ready and able to
approach forms of therapy or moves towards recovery, but that many others are not in
this position and may hence require a supportive environment in which to articulate
various narratives, which they may be unable to construct elsewhere.
2 Discourses such as these have typically been found to depoliticize the role that social
determinants of ill health may play.
3 Nevertheless, this does raise some issues that seem to be unresolved in literature of
online research ethics, in terms of protecting anonymity. It is possible that one might
search for the web pages by using the verbatim quotes found in our chapter. Since the
text is already within the public domain, this is not considered to be problematic,
although it does raise wider questions about the capacity to protect those using online
forums in research projects.
4 Saukko (2000) provides an interesting discussion on these tensions between discourse
and voice.

9 The bioethics of cybermedicalization

1 Indeed, the convergence of these areas is made evident by the existence of both scholarly studies of and political will to support work on the 'public engagement with ethics'
(see Miah 2005). Ashcroft (2003) describes this as the 'empirical turn' within bioethics.
2 For more general ethics and social science papers see the September 2006 issue of
Sociology of Health and Illness.
3 Thanks to James Auger for sharing this story at one of the Royal College of Art's
Design Interactions sessions in October 2006.
4 This is reminiscent of Žižek's story about the filming of 'David Lean's *Doctor Zhivago* in
a Madrid suburb in 1964'. As part of the performance, local inhabitants were gathered to
'sing the "Internationale" in a scene of mass demonstration' (Žižek 2004: xii). The happening developed to a point where other residents thought it genuine and believed that it
signalled the fall of Franco. As Žižek writes, 'these magic moments of illusory freedom'
constitute what we articulate here as the 'reality of the virtual' (ibid.: 3).
5 Indeed, the bioethics community can be quite neatly divided into those who accept this
premise and try to rewrite ethics on this basis, and those who contest it.
6 For examples of this broader digital paradigm through which to understand emerging
technology, see Nayar (2004).
7 One might also invoke the concept of 'public sociology' (Burawoy, cited in Brewer
2007: 176) as indicative of this trend within the social sciences to address future
issues. Delanty (2002) also makes explicit this problematic by noting that, in the context of genetics, 'scientific knowledge must be mediated by civic cultures of
knowledge' (p. 288).
8 While this work might seem distant from the pioneering anthropological work of the
twentieth century, Pfohl (1997) notes that Mead, Parsons, Bateson attended the
Macy Conferences, which themselves were discussions about undetermined future
societies.

9 The same claim we would make about the Gunther von Hagens' Body Worlds exhibits and his public autopsy in London during 2003 specifically (Miah 2004).

10 An alternative 'mundane cyborg' is articulated by Peterson (2007). This emphasizes the everyday function of the Internet in a way that is analogous to other household machines, such as refrigerators and coffee makers.

11 Indeed, at NYU in 2006, Haraway made explicit her rejection of this kind of posthumanism, which she more precisely wants to replace with 'ahumanism' a la Bruno Latour (personal communication, 2007, see also Haraway 2006b).

12 As Sobchack (2006) notes when discussing the prosthetic of below-the-knee amputee athlete/actress/model Aimee Mullins: the legs 'confuse such categories as human and animal and animate and inanimate in precisely the ironic way that Donna Haraway's cyborg was originally meant to do' (p. 35).

13 It is interesting to note that Zylinska's chapter on bioethics is titled '*Bio-ethics and cyberfeminism*', thus unavoidably being drawn into questions raised by Žižek in his 'Against hyper-ethics' (2004: 123). Zylinska's use of italics within her title suggests a similar concern about making ethics provisional in an era where new technology appears to raise new ethical questions, if not new ethical theories.

14 In more detail, Callahan notes the rise of bioethics in the United States as connected to liberal ideology. Perhaps the increasing need for new horizons reveals something about politics within the United States, though this has no necessary bearing on other political contexts. However, it is relevant to consider how the US approach to bioethics and medical ethics has informed other geographical regions.

Bibliography

Acton, M. and Spencer, R. (2006) 'I have 250 orgasms a day (and it's a scream)', *News of the World*, May 21, p. 45.

Allen, A. (2000) Morphing Telemedicine – Telecare – Telehealth – Ehealth. *Telemed Today*, Special Issue: Buyer's Guide and Directory (1): 43.

Aphramor, L. (2005) 'Is a weight-centred health framework salutogenic? Some thoughts on unhinging certain dietary ideologies.' *Social Theory and Health* 3: 315–40.

Armstrong, R. (2006) Multi-sectoral Health Promotion and Public Health: The Role of Evidence. *Journal of Public Health* 28(2): 168–72.

Armstrong, R., Doyle, J., Lamb, C., and Waters, E. (2006) Multi-sectoral health promotion and public health: the role of evidence, *Journal of Public Health* 2: 168–72.

Ashcroft, R. (2003) Constructing Empirical Bioethics: Foucauldian Reflects on the Empirical Turn in Bioethics Research. *Health Care Analysis* 11(1): 3–13.

Ashton, J. and Seymour, H. (1988) *The New Public Health*. Milton Keynes: Open University Press.

Aycock, A. (1993) Virtual Play: Baudrillard Online. *Electronic Journal of Virtual Culture* 1.

Bader, S. A. and Braude, R. M. (1998) 'Patient informatics': Creating new partnerships in medical decision making. *Academic Medicine* 73, 408–11.

Ballard, K. and Elston, M. (2005) Medicalisation: A Multi-dimensional Concept, *Social Theory and Health* (3): 228–41.

Balsamo, A. (1996/2000) The Virtual Body in Cyberspace. In D. Bell and B. Kennedy (eds) *The Cybercultures Reader*. Routledge: London. pp. 489–503.

Bandura, A. (1995) *Self-Efficacy: The Exercise of Control*. New York: W. H. Freeman.

Banthin, C., Blanke, D. and Archard, J. (2004). Legal Approaches to Regulating Internet Tobacco Sales. *Journal of Law, Medicine and Ethics* 32(S4): 64–8.

Barlow, J. P. (1996) A Declaration of the Independence of Cyberspace: http://hobbes.ncsa. uiuc.edu/sean/declaration.html.

Barnes, M. D., Penrod, C., Neiger, B. L., Merrill, R. M., Thackeray, R., Eggett, D. L. and Thomas, E. (2003) Measuring the Relevance of Evaluation Criteria among Health Information Seekers on the Internet. *Journal of Health Psychology* 8(1): 71–82.

Barney, S. (2005) Accessing Medicalized Donor Sperm in the US and Britain: An Historical Narrative. *Sexualities* 8(2): 205–20.

Barry, C., Bradley, P., Britten, N., Stevenson, F. and Barber, N. (2000) Patients' Unvoiced Agendas in General Practice Consultation: Qualitative Study. *British Medical Journal* 320(7244): 1246–1250.

Bassett, E. H. and O'Riordan, K. (2002) Ethics of Internet Research: Contesting the Human Subjects Research Model. *Ethics and Information Technology* 4: 233–47.

Bauer, K. A. (2001) Home-Based Telemedicine: A Survey of Ethical Issues. *Cambridge Quarterly of Healthcare Ethics* 10: 137–46.

Bauer, K. A. (2004) Cybermedicine and the Moral Integrity of the Physician–Patient Relationship. *Ethics and Information Technology* 6: 83–91.

Bauerle Bass, S. (2003). How Will Internet Use Affect the Patient? A Review of Computer Network and Closed Internet-Based System Studies and the Implications in Understanding How the Use of the Internet Affects Patient Populations. *Journal of Health Psychology* 8(1): 25–38.

BBC (1999) The First Human Clone. *Panorama.* UK, BBC1 (television programme).

BBC (2007) Outcry over TV Kidney Competition. Available at http://News.bbc.co.uk/1/Hi/Entertainment/6699847.Stm.

BBC Online (1999 (25 October)). World: America's Anger Greets Online Egg Auction: Hypertext Article. Available Online at: http://news2.thls.bbc.co.uk/hi/english/world/americas/newsid%5F483000/483784.stm.

Beck, U. (1992) From Industrial Society to Risk Society: Questions of Survival, Social Structure and Ecological Enlightenment. In M. Featherstone (ed.), *Cultural Theory and Cultural Change.* London: Sage.

Beck, U. and Beck-Gernsheim, E. (2002) *Individualization.* London: Sage.

Bereson, E. V., Gordon, C. and Herzog, D. B. (1989) The Process of Recovering from Anorexia Nervosa. *Journal of the American Academy of Psychoanalysis* 17: 103–30.

Berland, G. C., Elliott, M. N., Morales, L. S., Algazy, J. I., Kravitz, R. L., Broder, M. S. *et al.* (2001) Health Information on the Internet: Accessibility, Quality, and Readability in English and Spanish. *Journal of the American Medical Association* 285(20): 2612–2621.

Bernstein, B. (1990) Class, Codes and Control, vol. 4, *The Structuring of Pedagogic Discourse.* London: Routledge.

Bernstein, B. (1996) Class, Codes and Control, vol. 5, *Pedagogy, Symbolic Control and Identity: Theory, Research, Critique.* London: Taylor and Francis.

Bernstein, B. (1999) Vertical and Horizontal Discourse: An Essay. *British Journal of Sociology of Education* 20(2): 157–173.

Bernstein, B. (2001a) From Pedagogies to Knowledges. In A. Morais, I. Neves, B. Davies and H. Daniels (eds) *Towards a Sociology of Pedagogy: The Contribution of Basil Bernstein to Research.* New York: Peter Lang. pp. 363–368.

Bernstein, B. (2001b) Video Conference with Basil Bernstein. In A. Morais, I. Neves, B. Davies and H. Daniels (eds) *Towards a Sociology of Pedagogy: The Contribution of Basil Bernstein to Research.* New York: Peter Lang.

Biermann, J. S., Golladay, G. J., Greenfield, M. L. V. H. and Baker, L. H. (1999) Evaluation of Cancer Information on the Internet. *Cancer* 86: 381–390.

Biocca, F. (1997) The Cyborg's Dilemma: Progressive Embodiment in Virtual Environments. *Journal of Computer-Mediated Communications* 3(2): http://www.ascusc.org/jcmc/Vol3/Issue2/Biocca2.html.

Biressi, A. (2004) 'Above the Below': Body Trauma as Spectacle in Social/Media Space. *Journal for Cultural Research* 8: 335–352.

Bischoff, W. R. and Kelley, S. J. (1999) 21st Century House Call: The Internet and the World Wide Web. *Holistic Nursing Practice* 13(4): 42–50.

Blaxter, M. (1983) The Causes of Disease: Women Talking. *Social Science and Medicine* 17(2): 59–69.

Blaxter, M. (1997) Whose Fault Is It? People's Own Conceptions of the Reasons for Health Inequalities. *Social Science and Medicine* 44(6): 747–756.

Blum, J. D. (2003) Internet Medicine and the Evolving Legal Status of the Physician–Patient Relationship. *Journal of Legal Medicine* 24: 413–455.

Bonnickson, A. L. (1997) Procreation by Cloning: Crafting Anticipatory Guidelines. *Journal of Law, Medicine and Ethics* 25: 273.

Borowitz, S. M. and Wyatt, J. C. (1998) The Origin, Content, and Workload of E-Mail Consultations, *Journal of the American Medical Association* 280(15): 1321–1324.

Boseley, S. (2000) 'Virtual Healing: Life Online', Guardian Unlimited, 18 January. Online. Available: http://lifeonline.guardianunlimited.co.uk/week/story/0,6488,123729,00. htm.

Bouchard, C. (2000) Introduction. In C. Bouchard (ed.) *Physical Activity and Health.* Champaign, IL: Human Kinetics.

Boyd, J. (2002) In Community We Trust: Online Security Communication at eBay. *Journal of Computer-Mediated Communication* 7.

Braidotti, R. (2002) *Metamorphoses: Towards a Materialist Theory of Becoming,* Cambridge: Polity Press.

Brann, M. and Anderson, J. G. (2003) E-Medicine and Health Care Consumers: Recognizing Current Problems and Possible Resolutions for a Safer Environment. *Health Care Analysis* 10: 403–415.

Brewer, J. D. (2007) Review: *The New Sociological Imagination* by Steve Fuller. *European Journal of Social Theory* 10: 173–176.

British Medical Journal (1999) Editorial Paternalism or Partnership? *British Medical Journal* 319: 719–720.

Broom, D. H. (2001) Reading Breast Cancer: Reflections on a Dangerous Intersection. *Health* 5(2): 249–268.

Broom, D. H. and Woodward, R. V. (1996) Medicalization Reconsidered: Toward a Collaborative Approach to Care. *Sociology of Health and Illness* 18: 357–378.

Brown, J. (2001) 'The Winner Dies': A Web-Based Pro-Anorexia Movement Provides a Bizarre Support Network for Starving Girls, *Salon.Com*: http://archive.salon.com/ mwt/feature/2001/07/23/pro_ana/index_np.html.

Brownell, K. D. (1995) Definition and Classification of Obesity. In K. D. Brownell and C. G. Fairburn (eds) *Eating Disorders and Obesity: A Comprehensive Handbook.* New York: Guilford Press.

Bruckman, A. (2001) Ethical Guidelines for Research Online: A Strict Interpretation. http://www.cc.gatech.edu/~asb/ethics/.

Bryan, J. (2003) *Designer Vaginas.* UK, Channel 4 (television programme).

Bunton, R. and Burrows, R. (1995) Consumption and Health in the 'Epidemiological' Clinic of Late Modern Medicine. In R. Bunton, S. Nettleton and R. Burrows (eds) *The Sociology of Health Promotion.* London: Routledge.

Bunton, R. (1997) Popular Health, Advance Liberalism and Good Housekeeping. In A. Petersen and R. Bunton (eds) *Foucault, Health and Medicine.* New York: Routledge. pp. 223–248.

Burgermeister, J. (2004) UN Warns of Dangers of Drugs Sold on Internet. *British Medical Journal* 328(7440): 603.

Burkell, J. (2004) Health Information Seals of Approval: Why Do They Signify? *Information, Communication and Society* 7: 491–509.

Burrows, R., Nettleton, S., Pleace, N., Loader, B. and Muncer, S. (2000) Virtual Community Care? Social Policy and the Emergence of Computer Mediated Social Support. *Information, Communication and Society* 3(1): 95–121.

Burrows, L., and Wright, J. (2006) Prescribing Practices: Shaping Healthy Children in Schools, paper presented at 'Children and Young People as Social Actors' symposium, University of Otago.

Bury, M. (1982) Chronic Illness as Biographical Disruption. *Sociology of Health and Illness* 4: 167–182.

Bury, M. (1991) The Sociology of Chronic Illness: A Review of Research and Prospects. *Sociology of Health and Illness* 13: 451–468.

Bury, M. (2001) Illness Narratives: Fact or Fiction? *Sociology of Health and Illness* 23(3): 263–285.

Butler, J. (1993) *Bodies That Matter: On the Discursive Limits of 'Sex'*. London: Routledge.

Callahan, D. (1993) Why America Accepted Bioethics. *Hastings Center Report* 23: S8–S9.

Callahan, D. (1998) Cloning: Then And Now. *Cambridge Quarterly of Healthcare Ethics* 7: 141–144.

Calnan, M. And Gabe, J. (1991) Recent Developments in General Practice. In J. Gabe, M. Calnan and M. Bury (eds) *The Sociology of the Health Service*. London: Routledge.

Calvano, M. (1996) Public Empowerment through Accessible Health Information. *Bulletin of the Medical Library Association* 84(2): 253–256.

Campbell, S. (2006) Don't Tear a Smiling Foetus from the Womb. *The Telegraph* (London).

Campos, P. (2004) *The Obesity Myth*, Gotham Books.

Cant, S. and Sharma, U. (1999) *A New Medical Pluralism? Alternative Medicine, Doctors, Patients and the State*. London, UCL Press.

Caplan, A. (2004) Organs.Com: New Commercially Brokered Organ Transfers Raise Questions. *Hastings Center Report* 8.

Carpenter, K., Watson, J., Rafferty, B. and Chabal, C. (2003) Teaching Brief Interventions for Smoking Cessation via an Interactive Computer-Based Tutorial. *Journal of Health Psychology* 8(1): 149–160.

Cartwright, L. (1997) The Visible Man: The Male Criminal Subject as Biomedical Norm. In J. Terry and M. Calvert (eds) *Processed Lives: Gender and Technology in Everyday Life*. London: Routledge. pp. 123–137.

Castel, R. (1991) From Dangerousness to Risk. In G. Burchell, C. Gordon and P. Miller (eds) *The Foucault Effect: Studies in Governmentality*. London: Harvester Wheatsheaf.

Castell, M. (1996) The Information Age: Society and Culture, vol. 1, *The Rise of the Network Society*. Oxford: Blackwell Publishers.

Chen, X. and Siu, L. L. (2001) Impact of the Media and the Internet on Oncology: Survey of Cancer Patients and Oncologists in Canada. *Journal of Clinical Oncology* 19(23): 4291–4297.

Chesher, C. (1997) The Ontology of Digital Domains. In D. Holmes (ed.) *Virtual Politics: Identity and Community in Cyberspace*. London: Sage.

Chesley, E. B., Alberts, J. D., Klein, J. D. and Kreipe, R. E. (2003) Pro or Con? Anorexia Nervosa and the Internet. *Journal of Adolescent Health* 32: 123–124.

Cheung, C. (2004) Identity Construction and Self-Presentation on Personal Homepages: Emancipatory Potentials and Reality Constraints. In D. Gauntlett and R. Horsley (eds) *Web.Studies*, (2nd edition). London: Arnold.

Childress, C. A. (2000) Ethical Issues in Providing Online Psychotherapeutic Interventions. *Journal of Medical Internet Research* 2(1): E5.

China Internet Network Information Center (2007) Statistical Survey Report on the Internet Development in China.

Clarke, G. (1998) *Voices from The Margins: Lesbian Teachers in Physical Education.* Unpublished Doctoral Thesis. Leeds Metropolitan.

Clarke A. E. and Olsen, V. (1999) Revising, Diffracting, Acting. In A. E. Clarke and V. L. Olesen (eds) *Revisioning Women, Health and Healing: Feminist, Cultural and Technoscience Perspectives.* New York: Routledge. pp. 3–48.

Clarke, A. E., Mamo, L., Fishman, J. R., Shim, J. K. and Foskett, J. R. (2003) Biomedicalization: Technoscientific Transformations of Health, Illness and US Biomedicine. *American Sociological Review* 68: 161–194.

Clayton, L. (1997) Are There Virtual Communities? *Ends and Means: Journal of the University of Aberdeen Centre for Philosophy, Technology, and Society* 2. Available at http://www.abdn.ac.uk/philosophy/endsandmeans/vol2no1/clayton.shtml.

Cline, R. J. W. and Haynes, K. M. (2001) Consumer Health Information Seeking on the Internet: The State of the Art. *Health Education Research* 16: 671–692.

Cogan, J. (1999) Re-evaluating the Weight-Centered Approach toward Health: The Need for a Paradigm Shift. In J. Sobal and D. Maurer (eds) *Interpreting Weight: The Social Management of Fatness and Thinness.* New York: Aldine de Gruyter. pp. 229–254.

Cohen, J. C. (2004) Pushing the Borders: The Moral Dilemma of International Internet Pharmacies. *Hastings Center Report* 34: 15–17.

Coiera, E. (1996) The Internet's Challenge to Health Care Provision. *British Medical Journal* 312: 3–4.

Coiera, E. (1998) Information Epidemics, Economics, and Immunity on the Internet: We Still Know So Little about the Effect of Information on Public Health. *British Medical Journal* 317: 1469–1470.

Collste, G. (2002) The Internet Doctor and Medical Ethics: Ethical Implications of the Introduction of the Internet into Medical Encounters. *Medicine, Health Care and Philosophy* 5: 121–125.

Commission of the European Communities (2002) eEurope 2002: Quality Criteria for Health Related Websites. *Journal of Medical Internet Research* 4(3): e15.

Condit, C. M. and Williams, M. J. (1997) Audience Responses to the Discourse of Medical Genetics: Evidence against the Critique of Medicalization. *Health Communication* 9: 219–236.

Conrad, P. (1992) Medicalization and Social Control. *Annual Review of Sociology* 18: 209–232.

Conrad, P. (2005) The Shifting Engines of Medicalization. *Journal of Health and Social Behavior* 46: 3–14.

Conrad, P. and Schneider, J. W. (1980) *Deviance and Medicalization: From Badness to Illness.* St Louis: C. V. Mosby.

Cook, J. E. and Doyle, C. (2002) Working Alliance in Online Therapy as Compared to Face-to-Face Therapy: Preliminary Results. *CyberPsychology and Behavior* 5: 95–105.

COR Health care Resources (2001) Tipping the Scales: How the Net May Create a More Balanced Doctor–Patient Relationship. *Medicine on the Net* 7(5): 1–5.

Cordell, G. and Ronai, C. R. (1999) Identity Management among Overweight Women: Narrative Resistance to Stigma. In J. Sobal and D. Maurer (eds) *Interpreting Weight: The Social Management of Fatness and Thinness.* New York: Aldine de Gruyter. pp. 29–48.

Cornford, T. and Klecun-Dabrowska, E. (2001) Ethical Perspectives in Evaluation of Telehealth. *Cambridge Quarterly of Healthcare Ethics* 10: 161–169.

Coyle, A. and Sykes, C. (1998) Troubled Men and Threatening Women: The Construction of Crisis in Male Mental Health. *Feminism and Psychology* 8: 263–284.

Coyle, F. (2006) Posthuman Geographies? Biotechnology, Nature and the Demise of the Autonomous Human Subject. *Social and Cultural Geography* 7: 505–523.

Crawford, R. (1980) Healthism and the Medicalization of Everyday Life. *International Journal of Health Services* 10(3): 365–389.

Crawford, R. (1994) The Boundaries of the Self and the Unhealthy Other: Reflections on Health, Culture and AIDS. *Social Science and Medicine* 38(10): 1347–1365.

Croissant, J. L. (2006) The New Sexual Technobody: Viagra in the Hyperreal World. *Sexualities* 9: 333–344.

Cronenberg, D. (1986) *The Fly*, produced by Stuart Cornfeld (film).

Crossley, M. L. (2000) *Rethinking Health Psychology.* Buckingham, UK: Open University Press.

Crossley, M. (2001) Resistance and Health Promotion. *Health Education Journal* 60(3): 197–204.

Crossley, M. (2002) Resistance to Health Promotion and the 'Barebacking' Backlash. *Health* 6(1): 47–68.

Culver, J. D., Gerr, F. and Frumkin, H. (1997) Medical Information on the Internet: A Study of an Electronic Bulletin Board. *Journal of General Internal Medicine* 12: 466–470.

Cummins, C. O., Prochaska, J. O., Driskell, M. M., Kerry, E. E., Wright, J. A., Prochaska, J. M. and Velicer, W. F. (2003) Development of Review Criteria to Evaluate Health Behavior Change Websites. *Journal of Health Psychology* 8(1): 55–62.

Czaja, R., Manfredi, C., Price, J. (2003) The determinants and Consequences of Information Seeking Amongst Cancer Patients. *Journal of Health Communication* 8: 529–562.

David, M. (2005) *Science in Society.* Basingstoke, UK: Palgrave Macmillan.

Davis, L. (2006) Stumped by Genes: Lingua Gataca, DNA, and Prosthesis. In M. Smith and J. Morra (eds) *The Prosthetic Impulse: From a Posthuman Present to a Biocultural Future.* Cambridge, MA: MIT Press. pp. 91–106.

Davison, K. P., Pennebaker, J. W. and Dickerson, S. S. (2000) Who Talks? The Social Psychology of Illness Support Groups. *American Psychologist* 55(2): 205–217.

Delanty, G. (2002) Constructivism, Sociology and the New Genetics. *New Genetics and Society* 21(3): 279–289.

Department of Health (1998) *Information for Health: An Information Strategy for the Modern NHS*, 1998–2005. London: Department of Health.

Department of Health (1998) *Our Healthier Nation.* London: HMSO.

Department of Health (2001a) *Building the Information Core: Implementing the NHS Plan.* London: Department of Health.

Department of Health (2001b) First Patients Get On-Line Access to Their Own Medical Records: Pilot Trials Begin at Two GP Practices, press release, 21 January.

Department of Health (2003) *A Vision for Pharmacy in the New NHS.*

Dery, M. (1996) *Escape Velocity: Cyberculture at the End of the Century.* New York: Grove Press.

Devoss, D. (2000) Reading Cyborg Women: The Visual Rhetoric of Images of Cyborg (and Cyber) Bodies on the World Wide Web. *CyberPsychology and Behavior* 3: 835–845.

De Vries, R., Turner, L., Orfali, K. and Bosk, C. (2006) Social Science and Bioethics: The Way Forward. *Sociology of Health and Illness* 28: 665–677.

Dias, K. (2003) The Ana Sanctuary: Women's Pro-Anorexia Narratives in Cyberspace. *Journal of International Women's Studies* 4(2): 31–45.

Dibbell, J. (1993) A Rape in Cyberspace or How an Evil Clown, a Haitian Trickster Spirit, Two Wizards, and a Cast of Dozens Turned a Database into a Society. Available at http://www.juliandibbell.com/texts/bungle.html.

Dijck, J. V. (2000) Digital Cadavers: The Visible Human Project as Anatomical Theater. *Studies in History and Philosophy of Science* 31: 271–285.

Dijck, J. V. (2002) Medical Documentary: Conjoined Twins as a Mediated Spectacle. *Media, Culture, and Society* 24: 537–556.

Dixon-Woods, M. (2001) Writing Wrongs? An Analysis of Published Discourses about the Use of Patient Information Leaflets. *Social Science and Medicine* 52: 1417–1432.

Dobson, R. (2004) Meet Rudy, The World's First 'Robodoc'. *British Medical Journal* 329: 474.

Dodson, M. and Williamson, R. (1999) Indigenous Peoples and the Morality of the Human Genome Diversity Project. *Journal of Medical Ethics* 25: 204–208.

Dolan, D. (2003) Learning to Love Anorexia? 'Pro-Ana' Web Sites Flourish. *The New York Observer.* Available at http://www.observer.com/pages/story.asp?Id=6913.

Donath, J. S. (1996) Identity and Deception in the Virtual Community. In P. Kollock and K. Smith (eds) *Communities in Cyberspace.* London: Routledge. Available at http://smg.media.mit.edu/people/judith/identity/identitydeception.html.

Douglas, M. (1965) *Purity and Danger.* London: Routledge.

Dunham, P. J., Hurshman, A., Litwin, E., Gusella, J., Ellsworth, C. and Dodd, P. W. D. (1998) Computer-Mediated Social Support: Single Young Mothers as a Model System. *American Journal of Community Psychology* 26(2): 281–306.

Draper, H. (2000). 'Anorexia Nervosa and Respecting a Refusal of Life-Prolonging Therapy: A Limited Justification.' *Bioethics* 14(2): 120–133.

Dyer, K. A. (2001) Ethical Challenges of Medicine and Health on the Internet: A Review. *Journal of Medical Internet Research* 3: E23.

Eaton, L. (2002) Europeans and Americans Turn to Internet for Health Information. *British Medical Journal* 325: 989.

Ebrahim, D. W. (2002) Traumatic Separation Theory and Personality Disorder. *European Journal of Clinical Hypnosis* 5(2): 34–42.

Edgley, C. and Brissett, D. (1990) Health Nazis and the Cult of the Perfect Body; Some Polemical Observations. *Symbolic Interaction* 3(2): 257–280.

Elliott, C. (2003) *Better than Well: American Medicine Meets the American Dream.* New York: W. W. Norton.

Eng, T. R. (2001) *The eHealth Landscape: A Terrain Map of Emerging Information and Communication Technologies in Health and Health Care.* Princeton, NJ: Robert Wood Johnson Foundation.

Ess, C. (2002) Introduction. *Ethics and Information Technology* 4: 177–188.

Evans, J. (2003) Physical Education and Health: A polemic or let them eat cake! *European Physical Education Review* 9(1): 87–101.

Evans, R., Edwards, A. and Elwyn, G. (2003a) The Future for Primary Care: Increased Choice for Patients. *Quality and Safety in Health Care* 12: 83–84.

Evans, J., Evans, B. and Rich, E. (2003b) The Only Problem is They Will Like Their Chips. Education and the discursive production of ill-health. *Pedagogy, Culture and Society*, 11(2): 215–241.

Evans, J., Rich, E. and Davies, B. (2004) The Emperor's New Clothes: Fat, Thin and Overweight. The Social Fabrication of Risk and Ill-health. *Journal of Teaching in Physical Education* 23(4) 372–391.

Evans, J., Rich, E., Davies, B. and Allwood, R. (2005) The Embodiment of Learning: What the Sociology of Education Doesn't Say about 'Risk' in Going to School. *International Studies in the Sociology of Education* 15(2): 129–149.

Evans, J., Rich, E., Davies, B. and Allwood, R. (2008) *Fat Fabrications: Education, Eating Disorders and Obesity Discourse.* Abingdon, UK: Routledge.

Evers, K. E., Prochaska, J. M., Prochaska, J. O., Driskell, M., Cummins, C. O. and Velicier, W. F. (2003) Strengths and Weaknesses of Health Behavior Change Programs on the Internet. *Journal of Health Psychology* 8: 63–70.

Eysenbach, G. (1999) Online Prescribing of Sildanefil (Viagra) on the World Wide Web. *Journal of Medical Internet Research* 1: E10.

Eysenbach, G. and Diepgen, T. L. (1998) Towards Quality Management of Medical Information on the Internet: Evaluation, Labelling, and Filtering of Information. *British Medical Journal* 317: 1496–1500.

Eysenbach, G. and Diepgen, T. L. (1999) Labeling and Filtering of Medical Information on the Internet. *Methods of Information in Medicine* 38: 80–88.

Eysenbach, G. and T. Diepgen (1999) Patients Looking for Information on the Internet and Seeking Teleadvice: Motivation, Expectations, and Misconceptions as Expressed in E-mails Sent to Physicians. *Archives of Dermatology* 135(2): 151–156.

Eysenbach, G. and Köhler, C. (2002) How Do Consumers Search For and Appraise Health Information on the World Wide Web? Qualitative Study Using Focus Groups, Usability Tests, and In-Depth Interviews. *British Medical Journal* 324: 573–577.

Eysenbach, G., Ryoung, S. A. E. and Diepgen, T. L. (1999) Shopping around the Internet Today and Tomorrow: Towards the Millennium of Cybermedicine. *British Medical Journal* 319: 1294.

Federal Trade Commission *Consumer Alert: Virtual 'Treatments' Can Be Real World Deceptions.* Washington, DC: Federal Trade Comission, June 1999. Available at www.ftc.gov/bcp/conline/pubs/alerts/mrclalrt.pdf.

Ferguson, T. (1997) Health Online and the Empowered Medical Consumer. *Journal of Quality Improvement* 23(5): 251–257.

Ferguson, T. (2002) From Patients to End Users: Quality of Online Patient Networks Needs More Attention than Quality of Online Health Information. *British Medical Journal* 324(7337): 555–556.

Fernsler, J. and Manchester, L. (1997) Evaluation of a Computer-Based Cancer Support Network. *Cancer Practice* 5(1): 46–51.

Ferreday, D. J. (2003) Unspeakable Bodies: Erasure and Embodiment in Pro-Ana Communities. *International Journal of Cultural Studies* 6(3): 277 – 295.

Field, D. (ed.) (1996) *Telemedicine: A Guide to Assessing Telecommunications for Health Care.* Washington, DC: National Academy Press.

Finn, J. and Banach, M. (2000) Victimization Online: The Down Side of Seeking Human Services for Women on the Internet. *CyberPsychology and Behavior* 3(2): 243–254.

Fiore, M. C., Bailey, W. C., Cohen, S. J., *et al.* (2000) *Treating Tobacco Use and Dependence. Clinical Practice Guideline,* June. Rockville, MD: US Department of Health and Human Services, Public Health Service.

Fitzpatrick, M. (2001) *The Tyranny of Health: Doctors and the Regulation of Lifestyle.* London: Routledge.

Fitzpatrick, T. (1999) Social Policy for Cyborgs. *Body and Society* 5(1): 93–116.

Flatley-Brennan, P. (1998) Computer Network Home Care Demonstration: A Randomized Trial in Persons Living with AIDS. *Computers in Biology and Medicine* 28: 489–508.

Flegal, K. M. (1999) The Obesity Epidemic in Children and Adults: Current Evidence and Research Issues. *Medicine and Science in Sports and Exercise* 31:S509–S514.

Fogel, J., Albert, S. M., Schnabel, F., Ditkoff, B. A. and Neugut, A. I. (2002) Internet Use and Social Support in Women With Breast Cancer. *Health Psychology* 21(4): 398–404.

Fornaciari, C. and Roca, M. (1999) The Age of Clutter: Conducting Effective Research Using the Internet. *Journal of Management Education* 23(6): 732–742.

Foubister, V. (2000) Developing Rules for the Web. *American Medical News*, 31 July, 43: 11–12. Available at http://www.ama-assm.org/sci-pubs/amnews/pick_00/prsa 0731. htm.

Foucault, M. (1973) *The Birth of the Clinic: An Archaeology of Medical Perception*, trans. A. M. Sheridan Smith. New York: Vintage Books, 1994.

Foucault, M. (1978) *The History of Sexuality*, vol.1, *An Introduction.* London: Allen Lane.

Foucault, M. (1979) Governmentality. *Ideology and Consciousness* 6: 5–22.

Foucault, M (1980) In C. Gordon (ed.) *Power/Knowledge: Selected Interviews and Other Writings 1972–1977.* New York: Pantheon Books.

Foucault, M. (1984) The Politics of Health in the Eighteenth Century. In P. Rabinow (ed.) *The Foucault Reader.* New York: Pantheon Books. pp. 76–100.

Foucault, M. (1988) Truth, Power, Self. In L. Martin, H. Gutman and P. Hutton (eds) *Technologies of the Self: A Seminar with Michel Foucault.* London: Tavistock. pp. 12–12.

Foucault, M. (1996) The Return of Morality. In S. Lotringer (ed.) *Foucault Live: (Interviews, 1961–1984).* New York: Semiotext(E).

Fox, N. (1999) Postmodern Reflections on 'Risk', 'Hazards' and Life Choices. In D. Lupton (ed.) *Risk and Sociocultural.* Cambridge: Cambridge University Press.

Fox, N. J., Ward, K. J. and O'Rourke, A. J. (2005a) The 'Expert Patient': Empowerment or Medical Dominance? The Case of Weight Loss, Pharmaceutical Drugs and the Internet. *Social Science and Medicine* 60: 1299–1309.

Fox, N., Ward, K. and O'Rourke, A. (2005b) Pro-Anorexia, Weight-Loss Drugs and the Internet: An 'Anti-recovery' Explanatory Model of Anorexia. *Sociology of Health and Illness* 27(2): 944–971.

Fox, S. and Fallows, D. (2003) *Internet Health Resources*, Pew Internet And American Life Project. Available at: http://www.pewinternet.org/reports/ pdfs/pip_health_report_july_2003.pdf.

Fox, S. and L. Rainie (2002) *Vital Decisions: How Internet Users Decide What Information to Trust When They or Their Loved Ones are Sick.* Washington, DC: Pew Internet and American Life Project.

Fox, S. (2006) Online Health Search 2006. Pew Internet and American Life Project. October 29, 2006.

Frank, A. W. (1995) *The Wounded Storyteller: Body, Illness, and Ethics.* Chicago: University of Chicago Press.

Frank, A. (1997) Illness as Moral Occasion: Restoring Agency to Ill People. *Health: An Interdisciplinary Journal for the Social Study of Health, Illness and Medicine* 1, 131–48.

Freemantle, N. and Hill, S. (2002) Medicalisation, Limits to Medicine, or Never Enough Money to Go Around? Spending on Preventive Treatments That Help a Few Is Unaffordable. *British Medical Journal* 324: 864–865.

Freidson, E. (1970) *Professional Dominance: The Social Structure of Medical Care.* Chicago: Aldine.

Freidson, E. (1975) *Profession of Medicine: A Study of the Sociology of Applied Knowledge.* New York: Dodd, Mead.

Fukuyama, F. (1999) Second Thoughts: The Last Man in a Bottle. *The National Interest*, Summer: 1–18.

Fukuyama, F. (2002) *Our Posthuman Future: Consequences of the Biotechnology Revolution*. London: Profile Books.

Fukuyama, F. and Furger, F. (2007) *Beyond Bioethics: A Proposal for Modernizing the Regulation of Human Biotechnologies*. Washington, DC: Paul H. Nitze School of Advanced International Studies.

Fuller, S. (2006) *The New Sociological Imagination*. London: Sage.

Furedi, F. (2004) Reflections on the Medicalization of Social Experience. *British Journal of Guidance and Counselling* 32(3): 413–415.

Furedi, F. (2006) Our Unhealthy Obsession with Sickness, *Spiked online*, March 2005.

Gagliardi, A. and Jadad, A. R. (2002) Examination of Instruments Used to Rate Quality of Health Information on the Internet: Chronicle of a Voyage with An Unclear Destination. *British Medical Journal* 324: 569–573.

Gard, M. and Wright, J. (2001) Managing Uncertainty: Obesity Discourses and Physical Education in a Risk Society. *Studies in Philosophy and Education* 20: 535–549.

Gard, M. and Wright, J. (2005) *The Obesity Epidemic: Science, Morality and Ideology*. London: Routledge.

Garry, A. (2001) Medicine and Medicalization: A Response to Purdy. *Bioethics* 15: 262–269.

Gastaldo, D. (1997) Is Health Education Good for You? Rethinking Health Education through the Concept of Bio-power. In A. Petersen and R. Bunton (eds), *Foucault, Health and Medicine*. London: Routledge. pp. 113–133.

Gerhardt, U. (1990) Qualitative Research on Chronic Illness: The Issue and the Story. *Social Science and Medicine* 30(11): 1149–1159.

Gibson, W. (1984) *Neuromancer*. New York: Ace.

Gillam, S. and Brooks, F. (eds) (2001) *New Beginnings: Towards Patient and Public Involvement in Primary Health Care*. London: King's Fund.

Gillett, J. (2003) Media Activism and Internet Use by People With HIV/AIDS, *Sociology of Health and Illness* 25(6): 608–624.

Giustini, D. (2005) How Google is Changing Medicine: A Medical Portal is the Logical Next Step. *British Medical Journal* 331: 1487–1488.

Goldsmith, J. (2000) How will the Internet Change our Health System? *Health Affairs* 19(1): 148–56.

Good, B. (1994) *Medicine, Rationality and Experience: An Anthropological Perspective*. Cambridge: Cambridge University Press.

Gordijn, B. (2006) Converging NBIC Technologies for Improving Human Performance: A Critical Assessment of the Novelty and the Prospects of the Project. *Journal of Law, Medicine and Ethics* 34(4): 726–732.

Grace, V. M. (1991) The Marketing of Empowerment and the Construction of the Health Consumer: A Critique of Health Promotion. *International Journal Health Services* 21(2): 329–343.

Gradstein, D. S., Hofman, M. S. and Reuben, Y. (1995) Health Promotion on the Internet. *Reviews of Health Promotion and Education Online* (previously *Internet Journal of Health Promotion*), 18 October. Available at http://www.rhpeo.org/ijhp-articles/1995/1/index.htm.

Graham, E. (1999) Cyborgs or Goddesses? Becoming Divine in a Cyberfeminist Age. *Information, Communication and Society* 2: 419–438.

Granovetter, M. S. (1973) The Strength of Weak Ties. *American Journal of Sociology* 78, 1360–1380.

Gray, C. H. (2002) *Cyborg Citizen: Politics in the Posthuman Age*. London: Routledge.

Green, E. E., Thompson, D. and Griffiths, F. (2002) Narratives of Risk: Women at Midlife, Medical 'Experts' and Health Technologies. *Health, Risk and Society* 4 (3), 273–286.

Griffiths, M. (2000) Excessive Internet Use: Implications for Sexual Behaviour. *CyberPsychology and Behavior* 3(4): 537–552.

Grol, R. (2001) Foreword to A. Edwards and G. Elwyn (eds) *Evidence-Based Patient Choice: Inevitable or Impossible?* Oxford: Oxford University Press.

Groskopf, B. (2005) The Failure of Bio-power: Interrogating the 'Obesity Crisis'. *Journal for the Arts, Sciences and Technology* 3: 41–47.

Grosz, E. (2001) *Architecture from the Outside: Essays on Virtual and Real Space.* Cambridge, MA: MIT Press.

Gustafson, D., Wise, R., Mctavish, F. and Taylor, J. (1993) Development and Pilot Evaluation of a Computer-Based Support System for Women with Breast Cancer. *Journal of Psychosocial Oncology* 11(4): 69–93.

Gustafson, D. H., Robinson, T. N., Ansley, D., Adler, L. and Brennan, P. F. (1999a) Consumers and Evaluation of Interactive Health Communication Applications. *American Journal of Preventive Medicine* 16(1): 23–9.

Gustafson, D., Hawkins, R., Boberg, E., Pingree, S., Serlin, R. E., Graziano, F., and Chan, C. L. (1999b) Impact of a Patient-Centered, Computer-Based Health Information/Support System. *American Journal of Preventive Medicine* 16(1): 1–9.

Guttman, N. (2000) *Public Health Communication Interventions: Values and Ethical Dilemmas.* Thousand Oaks, CA: Sage.

Haimes, E. (2002) What Can The Social Sciences Contribute to the Study of Ethics? Theoretical, Empirical and Substantive Considerations. *Bioethics* 16: 89–113.

Hall, K. (1996) Cyberfeminism. In S. C. Herring (ed.) *Computer-Mediated Communication: Linguistic, Social and Cross-Cultural Perspectives.* Amsterdam and Philadelphia: John Benjamins Publishing Company. pp. 147–170.

Halse, C. (2007) The Bio-citizen: Virtue Discourses, BMI and Responsible Citizenship. Paper presented at the Bio-pedagogies Conference, University of Wollongong, 25–27 January.

Haraway, D. (1985/1991) A Cyborg Manifesto: Science, Technology, and Socialist-Feminism in the Late Twentieth Century. *Simians, Cyborgs and Women: The Reinvention of Nature.* New York: Routledge.

Haraway, D. (1988) Situated Knowledges: The Science Question in Feminism as a Site of Discourse on the Privilege of Partial Perspective. *Feminist Studies* 14: 575–99.

Haraway, D. (2006a) *The Companion Species Manifesto.* Chicago, Prickly Paradigm Press.

Haraway, D. (2006b) When we have never been human, what is to be done? Interview with Donna Haraway, *Theory, Culture and Society* 23(7–8): 135–158.

Hardey, M. (1999) Doctor in the House: The Internet as a Source of Lay Health Knowledge and the Challenge to Expertise. *Sociology of Health and Illness* 21: 820–835.

Hardey, M. (2001) 'E-Health': The Internet and the Transformation of Patients into Consumers and Producers of Health Knowledge. *Information, Communication and Society* 4: 388–405.

Hardey, M. (2002) 'The Story of My Illness': Personal Accounts of Illness on the Internet. *Health: An Interdisciplinary Journal for the Social Study of Health, Illness and Medicine* 6: 31–46.

Harlow, J. and Gould, M. (1999) Parents Target Oxbridge Egg Donors. *Sunday Times.* London. p. 12.

Harris, J. (1998) *Clones, Genes, and Immortality.* Oxford: Oxford University Press.

Harris, R. (1999) Come up to Beauty. Come up to Ron's Angels. 1999. Hypertext document. Available: http://www.ronsangels.com (Last accessed 12 June, 2007).

Harris Interactive (2001). Cyberchondriacs Update. The Harris Poll No.19. Harris Poll Library. Available at http://www.harrisinteractive.com/harris_poll/index.asp?pid=229 (accessed 11 March 2002).

Hart, A., Henwood, F., and Wyatt, S. (2003) The Role of the Internet in Mediating Relationships Between Patients and Practitioners: Hype and Reality. Conference discussion paper. Making Sense of Health, Illness and Disease Conference, St Hilda's College, Oxford 11–14 July.

Hartley, H. (2006) The 'Pinking' of Viagra Culture: Drug Industry Efforts to Create and Repackage Sex Drugs for Women. *Sexualities* 9(3): 363–378.

Harwood, V. (2006) *Diagnosing 'Disorderly' Children: A Critique of Behaviour Disorder Discourses.* London: Routledge.

Harwood, V. and Rasmussenm, M. L. (2004) Studying Schools with an Ethic of Discomfort. In B. Baker and K. Heyning (eds) *Dangerous Coagulations? The Uses of Foucault in the Study of Education.* New York: Peter Lang.

Have, H. A. M. J. T. (2001) Genetics and Culture: The Geneticization Thesis. *Medicine, Health Care and Philosophy* 4: 295–304.

Hayles, N. K. (1999) *How We Became Posthuman: Virtual Bodies in Cybernetics, Literature, and Informatics.* London: University of Chicago Press.

Hazlet, T. K. and Bach, M. H. M. (2001) The Internet, Confidentiality and the Pharmacy.Coms. *Cambridge Quarterly of Healthcare Ethics* 10: 157–160.

Health On the Net Foundation (HON). HON Code of Conduct (HONcode) for Medical and Health Web Sites: Principles. Available at http://www.hon.ch/honcode/conduct.html (accessed 5 March 2001).

Hedgecoe, A. (1998) Geneticization, Medicalization and Polemics. *Medicine, Health Care and Philosophy* 1(3): 235–243.

Hedgecoe, A. M. (2004) Critical Bioethics: Beyond the Social Science Critique of Applied Ethics. *Bioethics* 18: 120–143.

Heffan, I. V. (1997) Copyleft: Licensing Collaborative Works in the Digital Age. *Stanford Law Review* 49: 1487–1521.

Heim, M. (1993) *The Metaphysics of Virtual Reality.* New York: Oxford University.

Helmreich, S. (2001) ARTIFICIAL LIFE, INC.: Darwin and Commodity Fetishism from Santa Fe to Silicon Valley. *Science as Culture* 10(4): 484–504.

Henwood, S. (2006) Health E-Citizenship? Sociotechnical Systems and Self Care. Penceil Workshop, London School of Economics, 11–12 December.

Henderson, S. and Petersen, A. (2002) Introduction: Consumerism in Health Care. In S. Henderson and A. Petersen (eds) *Consuming Health: The Commodification of Health Care.* London: Routledge.

Henson, D. E. (1999) Cancer and the Internet. *Cancer* 86: 373–374.

Henwood, F., Wyatt, S., Hart, A. and Smith, J. (2003) Ignorance Is Bliss Sometimes. *Sociology of Health and Illness* 25(6): 589–607.

Hersh, W. R. (1996) Evidence-Based Medicine and the Internet [editorial]. *ACP Journal Club* 125: A14–A16.

HON's Fourth Survey on the Use of the Internet for Medical and Health Purposes. Available at www.hon.ch/survey/resumeapr99.html (accessed 28 June 1999).

Higham, J. (2007) Ulrika. *Am I a Sex Addict?* Channel 4 (television programme).

Hine, C. (2000) *Virtual Ethnography.* London: Sage.

Hine, C. (2001) Web Pages, Authors and Audiences: The Meaning of a Mouse Click. *Information, Communication and Society* 4: 182–198.

Hodgetts, D. and Chamberlain, K. (1999) Medicalization and the Depiction of Lay People in Television Health Documentary. *Health* 3: 317–333.

Hodgetts, D. and Chamberlain, K. (2003) Television Documentary in New Zealand and the Construction of Doctors by Lower Socio-Economic Groups. *Social Science and Medicine* 57: 113–124.

Holmes, D. (1997) Virtual Identity: Communities of Broadcast, Communities of Interactivity. In D. Holmes (ed.) *Virtual Politics: Identity and Community in Cyberspace.* London: Sage.

Hong, T. and Cody, M. J. (2002) Presence of Pro-Tobacco Messages on the Web. *Journal of Health Communication* 7: 273–307.

Hsiung, R. C. (2000) The Best of Both Worlds: An Online Self-Help Group Hosted by a Mental Health Professional. *CyberPsychology and Behavior* 3(6): 935–950.

Human Genetics Advisory Commission (1998) *Cloning Issues in Reproduction, Science and Medicine,* December.

Huntley, (1999) The Need to Know: Patients, E-Mail and the Internet. *Archives of Dermatology* 135, 198–199.

Illich, I. (1975) *Limits to Medicine.* London: Marion Boyars.

Impicciatore, P., Pandolfini, C., Casella, N. and Bonati, M. (1997) Reliability of Health Information for the Public on the World Wide Web: Systematic Survey of Advice on Managing Fever in Children at Home. *British Medical Journal* 314: 1875–1881.

Jadad, A. R. (1999) Promoting Partnerships: Challenges for the Internet Age. *British Medical Journal* 319: 761–764.

Jadad, A. R. and Gagliardi, A. (1998) Rating Health Information on the Internet: Navigating to Knowledge or to Babel? *Journal of the American Medical Association* 279: 611–614.

Johnson, K., Ravert, R. and Everton, A. (2001) Hopkins Teen Central: Assessment of an Internet-Based Support System for Children with Cystic Fibrosis. *Pediatrics* 107(2): E24.

Jones, S. G. (ed.) (1995) *Cybersociety: Computer-Mediated Communication and Community.* London: Sage.

Jones, S. G. (1997a) The Internet and Its Social Landscape. In S. G. Jones (ed.) *Virtual Culture: Identity and Communication in Cybersociety.* London: Sage. pp. 7–35.

Jones, S. G. (ed.) (1997b) *Virtual Culture: Identity and Communication in Cybersociety.* London: Sage.

Juengst, E. T. (1998) What Does *Enhancement* Mean? In E. Parens (ed.) *Enhancing Human Traits: Ethical and Social Implications.* Washington, DC: Georgetown University Press. pp. 29–47.

Kahan, S. E., Seftel, D. and Resnik, M. I. (2000) Sildenafil and the Internet. *Journal of Urology* 163: 919–923.

Kassirer, J. P. and Angell, M. (1998) Losing Weight: An Ill-Fated New Year's Resolution. *New England Journal of Medicine* 338: 52–54.

Kedar, I., Ternullo, J. L., Weinrib, C. E., Kelleher, K. M., Branding-Bennett, H. and Kvedar, J. C. (2003) Information in Practice. *British Medical Journal* 326: 696–699.

Kellner, D. (2003) *Media Spectacle.* London: Routledge.

Kelly, K. (1994) *Out of Control: The New Biology of Machines.* London: Fourth Estate.

Kember, S. (1998) *Virtual Anxiety: Photography, New Technologies, and Subjectivity.* Manchester: Manchester University Press.

Kember, S. (1999) NITS And NRTS: Medical Science and the Frankenstein Factor. In Cutting Edge: The Women's Research Group (ed.) *Desire by Design: Body, Territories, and New Technologies*. London: I. B. Tauris.

Kennedy, B. (2000) Cyberbodies: Introduction. In D. Bell and B. Kennedy (eds) *The Cybercultures Reader*. London: Routledge. pp. 471–476.

Khrjanovsky, I. (dir.) (2005) *4*. Russia (film).

Kitchin, R. (1998) *Cyberspace: The World in Wires*. Chichester: John Wiley and Sons.

Kivits, J. (2004) Researching the 'Informed Patient'. *Information, Communication and Society* 7: 510–530.

Kleinman, A. (1988) *The Illness Narratives: Suffering, Healing and the Human Condition*. New York: Basic Books.

Komesaroff, P. (1995) From Bioethics to Microethics: Ethical Debate and Clinical Medicine. In Paul Komesaroff (ed.) *Troubled Bodies: Critical Perspectives on Postmodernism, Medical Ethics and the Body*. Durham, NC: Duke University Press. pp. 62–86.

Kraut, R., Patterson, M., Lundmark, V., Kiesler, S., Mukopadhyay, T. and Scherlis, W. (1998) Internet Paradox: A Social Technology That Reduces Social Involvement and Psychological Well-Being? *American Psychologist* 53: 1017–1031.

Kroker, A. and Kroker, M. (1987) Body Digest: Theses on the Disappearing Body in the Hyper-Modern Condition. *Canadian Journal of Political and Social Theory* 11: i–xvi.

Kroker, A. and Weinstein, M. (1994) The Hyper-Texted Body, or Nietzsche Gets a Modem. *CTHEORY*. Available at http://www.ctheory.net/articles.aspx?id=144.

Kroll-Smith, S. (2003) Popular Media and 'Excessive Daytime Sleepiness': A Study of Rhetorical Authority in Medical Sociology. *Sociology of Health and Illness* 25(6): 625–643.

Kvedar, J. C. (2003) Internet Based Consultations to Transfer Knowledge for Patients Requiring Specialised Care: Retrospective Case Review. *British Medical Journal* 326: 696–699.

Lancet, The (1998) Viagra's Licence and the Internet (editorial). *The Lancet*, 352: 751.

Lander, M. (2004) German Court Convicts Internet Cannibal of Manslaughter. *New York Times* (New York). Available at http://www.nytimes.com/2004/01/31/international /europe/31germ.html?ei=5007anden=b1d3ae530b3cc082andex=1390885200andparter =userlandandpagewanted=printandposition=.

Lask, B. and Bryant-Waugh, R. (eds) (2000) *Anorexia nervosa and related eating disorders in childhood and adolescence*. London: Taylor and Francis.

Leonard, B. (1992) *The Lawnmower Man*. Ben Jade Films Inc. (film).

Lewin, E. and Olesen, V. (eds) (1985) *Women, Health and Healing: Toward a New Perspective*. New York: Methuen/Tavistock.

Lewis, J. (2006) Making Order out of a Contested Disorder: The Utilisation of Online Support Groups in Social Science Research. *Qualitative Researcher* 3: 4–7.

Lewis, T. (2006) Seeking Health Information on the Internet: Lifestyle Choice or Bad Attack of Cybercchondria? *Media, Culture and Society* 28(4): 521–539.

Loader, B.D., Muncer, S., Burrows, R., Pleace, N. and Nettleton, S. (2002) Medicine on the Line? Computer-Mediated Social Support and Advice for People with Diabetes. *International Journal of Social Welfare* 11: 53–65.

Locke, M. (1998) Anomalous Ageing: Managing the Postmenopausal Body. *Body and Society* 4: 35–61.

Loe, M. (2004) *The Rise of Viagra: How the Little Blue Pill Changes Sex in America*. New York: New York University Press.

London Net (2007) David Hasselhoff Drunk-on-Tape Antics All Over the Internet. London Net. London. Available at http://www.londonnet.co.uk/entertainment/2007/may/5716_20070504.php (accessed 4 July 2007).

Longo, R. (1995) *Johnny Mnemonic*. USA (film).

López, J. (2004) How Sociology Can Save Bioethics. Maybe. *Sociology of Health and Illness* 26: 875–896.

Lowenberg, J. and Davis, F. (1994) Beyond Medicalisation–Demedicalisation: the Case of Holistic Health. *Sociology of Health and Illness* 16(5): 579–99.

Lund, J. (2002) My Personal PSAS Story: Persistent Sexual Arousal Syndrome: Is This a New Medical Phenomena Distressing Women? http://members.tripod.com/jeannie_allen/id40.htm (accessed 4 July 2007).

Lupton, D. (1995) *The Imperative of Health: Public Health and the Regulated Body*. London: Sage.

Lupton, D. (1997) Consumerism, Reflexivity and the Medical Encounter. *Social Science and Medicine* 45(3): 373–381.

Lupton, D. (1998) Foucault and the Medicalization Critique. In A. Petersen and R. Bunton (eds) *Foucault, Health and Medicine*. London: Routledge.

Lupton, D. (1999a) Editorial: Health, Illness, and Medicine in the Media. *Health: An Interdisciplinary Journal for the Social Study of Health, Illness and Medicine* 3: 259–262.

Lupton, D. (1999b) *Risk*. London: Routledge.

Lupton, D. (2003) *Medicine as Culture: Illness, Disease and the Body in Western Societies*. London: Sage.

Lynn, R. (2007) Virtual Rape Is Traumatic, but Is It a Crime? *Wired*. Available at http://www.wired.com/print/culture/lifestyle/commentary/sexdrive/2007/05/sexdrive_0504.

Lyons, A. C. (2000) Examining Media Representations: Benefits for Health Psychology. *Journal of Health Psychology* 5: 349–358.

Lyons, A. C. and Willott, S. (1999) From Suet Pudding to Superhero: Representations of Men's Health for Women. *Health* 3: 283–302.

McCarthy, H. and Miller, P. (2003) *London Calling: How Mobile Technologies Will Transform Our Capital City*. London: Demos.

Macintyre, M. (2003) Internet: Changing the Medical Encounter? Paper presented at the *Association of Internet Researchers Fourth Annual Conference*, Toronto, Ontario, 16–19 October. Available at http://kmi.open.ac.uk/people/macintyre/aoir2003paper.htm.

McKenna K. Y. A. and Bargh, J. A. (1999a) Causes and Consequences of Social Interaction on the Internet: A Conceptual Framework. *Media Psychology* 1: 249–269.

McKenna K. Y. A. and Bargh, J. A. (1999b) Coming Out in the Age of the Internet: Identity 'Demarginalization' through Virtual Group Participation. *Journal of Personality and Social Psychology* 75: 681–694.

MacKinnon, R. (1997) Virtual Rape. *Journal of Computer-Mediated Communication* 2(4). Available at http://jcmc.indiana.edu/vol2/issue4/mackinnon.html.

McLaughlin, J. (1975) The Doctor Shows. *Journal of Communication* 25: 182–184.

McLeod, S. (1998) The Quality of Medical Information on the Internet: A New Public Health Concern. *Archives of Ophthamology* 116: 1663–1665.

Mahowald, M. B. (1994) Reproductive Genetics and Gender Justice. In K. H. Rothenberg and E. J. Thomson (eds) *Women and Prenatal Testing: Facing the Challenges of Genetic Technology*. Columbus: Ohio State University.

Mainzer, K. (1998) Computer Technology and Evolution: From Artificial Intelligence to Artificial Life. *Techne: Society for Philosophy and Technology* 4(1): 105–118.

Makus, R. (2001) Ethics and Internet Health care: An Ontological Reflection. *Cambridge Quarterly of Healthcare Ethics* 10: 127–136.

Malson, H. (1998) *The Thin Woman: Feminism, Poststructuralism and the Social Pyschology of Anorexia Nervosa.* London: Routledge.

Mamo, L. (2007) Negotiating Conception: Lesbians' Hybrid-Technological Practices. *Science, Technology, and Human Values* 32: 369–393.

Mamo, L. and Fishman, J. R. (2001) Potency in All the Right Places: Viagra as a Technology of the Gendered Body. *Body and Society* 7(4): 13–35.

Mandl, K. D., Kohane, I. S. and Brandt, A. M. (1998) Electronic Patient–Physician Communication: Problems and Promise. *Annals of Internal Medicine* 129: 495–500.

Manhal-Baugus, M. (2001) E-Therapy: Practical, Ethical, and Legal Issues. *CyberPsychology and Behavior* 4(5): 551–563.

Mar, C. M., Chabal, C., Anderson, R. A. and Vore, A. E. (2003) An Interactive Computer Tutorial to Teach Pain Assessment. *Journal of Health Psychology* 8(1):161–173.

Marshall, B. L. (2002) 'Hard Science': Gendered Constructions of Sexual Dysfunction in the 'Viagra Age'. *Sexualities* 5(2): 131–158.

Marshall, B. L. (2006) The New Virility: Viagra, Male Aging and Sexual Function. *Sexualities* 9(3): 345–362.

Martin, J. (2004) The Educational Inadequacy of Conceptions of Self in Educational Psychology. *Interchange* 35(2) 185–208.

Marton, C. (2000) Evaluating the Women's Health Matters Website. *CyberPsychology and Behavior* 3(5): 747–759.

Massé, R., Legare, F., Cote, L. and Dodin, S. (2001) The Limitations of a Negotiation Model for Perimenopausal Women. *Sociology of Health and Illness* 23(1): 44–64.

Mathieson, C. M. and Stam, H. J. (1995) Renegotiating Identity: Cancer Narratives. *Sociology of Health and Illness* 17: 283–306.

Mechanic, D. (1999) Issues in Promoting Health. *Social Science and Medicine* 48(6): 711–718.

Melzer, D. and R. Zimmern (2002) Genetics and Medicalisation: Genetics Could Drive a New Wave of Medicalisation if Genetic Tests are Accepted Without Appropriate Clinical Evaluation. *British Medical Journal* 324: 863–864.

Metz, R. (2006) Lying Through Their Teeth. *Wired.* Available at http://www.wired.com/culture/lifestyle/news/2006/04/70601?currentpage=all.

Metzl, J. M. and Herzig, R. M. (2007) Medicalization in the 21st Century: Introduction. *The Lancet* 369: 697–698.

Miah, A. (2003) Patenting Human DNA. In B. Almond and M. Parker (eds) *Ethical Issues in the New Genetics.* Aldershot, UK: Ashgate. pp. 111–118.

Miah, A. (2004) The Public Autopsy: Somewhere Between Art, Education and Entertainment. *Journal of Medical Ethics* 30: 576–579.

Miah, A. (2005) Genetics, Cyberspace and Bioethics: Why Not a Public Engagement with Ethics? *Public Understanding of Science* 14(4): 409–421.

Miah, A. (2008) Posthumanism: A Critical History. In B. Gordijn and R. Chadwick (eds) *Medical Enhancements and Posthumanity.* London: Springer.

Miles, A. (1991) *Women, Health and Medicine.* Milton Keynes, UK: Open University Press.

Miller, T. and Reents, S. (1998) The Health Care Industry in Transition: The Online Mandate to Change. *Cyberdialogue.* Available at http://www.cyberdialogue.com/pdfs/white_papers/intel.pdf (accessed 13 August 1999).

Mitchell, W. J. (1995) *City of Bits: Space, Place, and the Infobahn*. Cambridge, MA: MIT Press.

Mitchell, J. (1999) *From Telehealth to e-Health: The Unstoppable Rise of e-Health* Canberra, Australia: National Office for the Information Economy.

Mitra, A. (1997) Virtual Commonality: Looking for India on the Internet. In S. G. Jones (ed.) *Virtual Culture: Identity and Communication in CyberSociety*. London: Sage. pp. 55–79.

Mitra, A. (2001) Marginal Voices in Cyberspace. *New Media and Society* 3: 29–48.

Mnookin, J. L. (1996) Virtual(ly) Law: The Emergence of Law in LambdaMOO. *Journal of Computer-Mediated Communication* 2(1). Available at http://jcmc.indiana. edu/vol2/issue1/lambda.html.

Monaghan, L. (2005) Discussion Piece: A Critical Take on the Obesity Debate. *Social Theory and Health* 3(4): 302–314.

Monks, J. (2000) Talk as Social Suffering: Narratives of Talk in Medical Settings. *Anthropology and Medicine* 7(1): 15–38.

Moore, M. (2007) *Sicko*. USA (film).

Morgentaler, A. (2003) *The Viagra Myth: The Surprising Impact on Love and Relationships*. San Francisco: Jossey-Bass.

Moynihan, R. and Smith, R. (2002) Too Much Medicine? Almost Certainly. *British Medical Journal* 324: 859–860.

Moynihan, R. (2003) The Making of a Disease: Female Sexual Dysfunction. *British Medical Journal* 326: 45–47.

Moynihan, R. I. Heath, I. and Henry, D. (2002) Selling Sickness: the Pharmaceutical Industry and Disease Mongering. *British Medical Journal* 324: 886–891.

Muir Gray, J. A (2002) *The Resourceful Patient*. Oxford: Erosetta Press.

Mules, W. (2000) Virtual Culture, Time and Images: Beyond Representation. *M/C: A Journal of Media and Culture* 3(2). Available at http://journal.media-culture.org.au/0005/images.php (accessed July 2003).

Murray, M. (1997) A Narrative Approach to Health Psychology. *Journal of Health Psychology* 2: 9–20.

Murray, M. (2000) Levels of Narrative Analysis in Health Psychology. *Journal of Health Psychology* 5: 337–347.

Nakamura, L. (2002) *Cybertypes: Race, Ethnicity, and Identity on the Internet*. London: Routledge.

Nash, K. (2001) The 'Cultural Turn' in Social Theory: Towards a Theory of Cultural Politics. *Sociology* 35: 77–92.

Nayar, P. K. (2004) *Virtual Worlds: Culture and Politics in the Age of Cybertechnology*. Delhi: Sage.

Nerlich, B. and Clarke, D.A. (2003) Anatomy of a Media Event: How Arguments Clashed in the 2001 Human Cloning Debate. *New Genetics and Society* 22(1): 43–59.

Nerlich, B., Johnson, S. and Clarke, D. D. (2003) The First 'Designer Baby': The Role of Narratives, Clichés and Metaphors in the Year 2000 Debate. *Science as Culture* 12: 471–498.

Nettleton, S. (1996) *The Sociology of Health and Illness*. Cambridge: Polity Press.

Nettleton, S. (1997) Governing the Risky Self: How to Become Healthy, Wealthy and Wise. In A. Petersen and R. Bunton (eds), *Foucault, Health and Medicine*. London: Routledge. pp. 207–222.

Nettleton, S. (2004) The Emergence of e-Scaped Medicine. *Sociology* 38: 661–679.

Nettleton, S. and Bunton, R. (1995) Sociological Critique of Health Promotion. In S. Nettleton, R. Bunton and R. Hampshire (eds) *The Sociology of Health Promotion.* London: Routledge.

Nettleton, S. and Burrows, R. (2003) E-Scaped Medicine? Information, Reflexibility and Health. *Critical Social Policy* 23: 165–185.

Nettleton, S., Burrows, R., O'Malley, L. and Watt, I. (2003) *Children, Parents and the Management of Chronic Illness in the Information Age.* London: Economic and Social Research Council, Innovative Health Technologies Programme.

Nettleton, S., Burrows, R., O'Malley, L. and Watt, I. (2004) Health E-Types? An Analysis of the Everyday Use of the Internet for Health. *Information, Communication and Society* 7: 531–553.

Nettleton, S., Burrows, R. and O'Malley, L. (2005) The Mundane Realities of the Everyday Lay Use of the Internet for Health, and Their Consequences for Media Convergence. *Sociology of Health and Illness* 27(7): 972–992.

Neuhauser, L. and G. Kreps, L. (2003) Rethinking communication in the E-health era. *Journal of Health Psychology* 8(1): 7–23.

NHS Executive (1996) *Patient Partnership: Building a Collaborative Strategy.* London: HMSO.

NHS Executive (1997) *The New NHS: Modern, Dependable.* London: The Stationery Office.

Nicholas, D., Huntington, P., Williams P. and Blackburn, P. (2001) Digital Health Information Provision and Health Outcomes. *Journal of Information Science* 27(4): 265–276.

O'Brien, M. (1995) Health and Lifestyle: A Critical Mess? Notes on the Dedifferentiation of Health. In R. Bunton, S. Nettleton and R. Burrows (eds) *The Sociology of Health Promotion.* London: Routledge.

O'Reilly, T. (2005) What is Web 2.0: Design Patterns and Business Models for the Next Generation of Software. O'Reilly Net: http://www.oreillynet.com/pub/a/oreilly/tim/news/2005/09/30/what-is-web-20.html (Accessed 8 July 2006).

Oliver, A. J. (2000) Internet Pharmacies: Regulation of a Growing Industry. *Journal of Law, Medicine and Ethics* 28: 98.

Oravec, J. A. (2000) On-Line Medical Information and Service Delivery: Implications for Health Education. *Journal of Health Education* 31: 105–109.

Orgad, S. (2004) Help Yourself: The World Wide Web as a Self-Help Agora. In D. Gauntlett and R. Hors (eds) *Web.Studies* (2nd edn). London: Arnold. pp. 147–157.

Pandey, S. K., Hart, J. J. and Tiwary, S. (2003) Women's Health and the Internet: Understanding Emerging Trends and Implications. *Social Science and Medicine* 56(1): 179–191.

Parker, M. and Muir Gray, J. A. (2001) What Is the Role of Clinical Ethics Support in the Era of E-Medicine? *Journal of Medical Ethics* 27, (Suppl. 1: I): 33–35.

Payne, S., Large, S., Jarrett, N. and Turner, P. (2000) Written Information Given to Patients and Families by Palliative Care Units: A National Survey. *The Lancet* 355: 1792.

Pence, G. E. (2000) *Re-creating Medicine: Ethical Issues at the Frontiers of Medicine.* Oxford: Rowman and Littlefield.

People's Daily Online (2007) 480 million Mobile Phone Users in China. *People's Daily Online.*

Petersen, A. (1996) Risk and the Regulated Self: The Discourse of Health Promotion as Politics of Uncertainty. *Australian and New Zealand Journal of Sociology* 33(1), 44–57.

Petersen, A. and Lupton, D. (1996) *The New Public Health: Health and Self in the Age of Risk.* London: Allen and Unwin; Sydney: Sage.

Peterson, S. M. (2007) Mundane Cyborg Practice: Material Aspects of Broadband Internet Use. *Convergence: The International Journal of Research into New Media Technologies* 13: 79–91.

Pew Internet and American Life Project (2000) *The Online Health Care Revolution: How the Web Helps Americans Take Better Care of Themselves.* Summary of Findings: The Internet's Powerful Influence on 'Health Seekers'. 26 November. Available at http://www.pewinternet.org/reports/toc.asp?report=26.

Pfohl, S. (1997) The Cybernetic Delirium of Norbert Wiener. *Ctheory*, 30 January. Available at http://www.ctheory.net/yext_gile.ssp?pick=86.

Pingree, S., Hawkins, R. P., Gustafson, D. H., Boberg, E., Bricker, E., Wise, M., Berhe, H. and Hsu, E. (1996) Will the Disadvantaged Ride the Information Highway? Hopeful Answers from a Computer-Based Health Crisis System. *Journal of Broadcasting and Electronic Media* 40(3): 331–353.

Pitts, V. (2004) Illness and Internet Empowerment: Writing and Reading Breast Cancer in Cyberspace. *Health: An Interdisciplinary Journal for the Social Study of Health, Illness and Medicine* 8: 33–59.

Pollack, D. (2003) Pro-Eating Disorder Websites: What Should Be the Feminist Response? *Feminism and Psychology* 13(2): 246–251.

Porter, R. (1998) *Health For Sale: Quackery in England, 1650–1850.* Manchester: Manchester University Press.

Poster, M. (1997) Cyberdemocracy: The Internet and the Public Sphere. In D. Holmes (ed.) *Virtual Politics: Identity and Community in Cyberspace.* London: Sage. pp. 212–228.

Potts, A. (2004) Deleuze on Viagra (or, What Can a 'Viagra-Body' Do?). *Body and Society* 10: 17–36.

Powell, J., McCarthy, N. and Eysenbach, G. (2003) Cross-sectional Survey of Users of Internet Depression Communities. *BMC Psychiatry* 3: 19. Published Online 10 December 2003. Available at http://www.pubmedcentral.nih.gov/articlerender.fcgi?artid=317315.

Prasad, A. (2005) Making Images/Making Bodies: Visibilizing and Disciplining through Magnetic Resonance Imaging (MRI). *Science, Technology, and Human Values* 30: 291–316.

Preece, J. J. and Ghozati, K. (2001) Experiencing Empathy Online. In R. E. Rice and J. E. Katz (eds) *The Internet and Health Communication.* Thousand Oaks, CA: Sage. pp. 237–260.

Purdy, L. (2001a) Medicalization, Medical Necessity, and Feminist Medicine. *Bioethics* 15: 248–261.

Purdy, L. M. (2001b) What Feminism Can Do for Bioethics. *Health Care Analysis* 9: 117–132.

Quinn, B. (2001) The Medicalisation of Online Behaviour. *Online Information Review* 25(3): 173–180.

R. v. Human Fertilisation and Embryology Authority, ex p. Blood [1997] 2 All ER 687; (1997) 35 BMLR 1 (CA).

Rabinow, P. and Rose, N. (2006) Biopower Today. *Biosocieties* 1: 195–217

Radley, A. (1994) *Making Sense of Illness: The Social Psychology of Health and Disease.* London: Sage.

Radley, A. (1999) The Aesthetics of Illness: Narrative, Horror and the Sublime. *Sociology of Health and Illness* 21: 778–796.

Rajagopal, S. (2004) Editorial: Suicide Pacts and the Internet. *British Medical Journal* 329: 1298–1299.

Reaves, J. (2001) Anorexia Goes High Tech. *Time*, 31 July. Available at http://www.time.com.

Reeves, P. (2001) How Individuals Coping with HIV/AIDS Use the Internet. *Health Education Research* 16: 709–719.

Resnik, D. B. (2001a) Patient Access to Medical Information in the Computer Age: Ethical Concerns and Issues. *Cambridge Quarterly of Healthcare Ethics* 10: 147–156.

Resnik, D. B. (2001b) Regulating the Market for Human Eggs. *Bioethics* 15: 1–25.

Rheingold, H. (1993) *The Virtual Community.* Reading, MA: Addison-Wesley.

Rice, R.E. and Katz, J. E. (2001) *The Internet and Health Communication: Experiences and Expectations.* Thousand Oaks, CA: Sage.

Rich, E. (2006) Anorexic (Dis)Connection. *Sociology of Health and Illness* 28(3): 284–305

Rich, E. and Evans, J. (2005) Making Sense of Eating Disorders in Schools. *Discourse: Studies in the Cultural Politics of Education* 26(2): 247–262.

Rich, E., Harjunen, H., and Evans, J. (2006) Normal Gone Bad – Health Discourses, Schools and the Female Body. In P. Twohig and V. Kalitzkus (eds) *Bordering Biomedicine Interdisciplinary Perspectives on Health, Illness and Disease.* Amsterdam: Rodopi Publications.

Richardson, K. P. (2003) Health Risks on the Internet: Establishing Credibility On Line. *Health, Risk and Society* 5(2): 171–184.

Risk, A. and Dzenowagis, J. (2001) Review of Internet Health Information Quality Initiatives. *Journal of Medical Internet Research* 3(4): E288.

Ritenbaugh, C. (1982) Obesity as a Culture Bound Syndrome. *Culture, Medicine and Psychiatry* 6: 348–361.

Robins, K. (1996/2000) Cyberspace and the World We Live In. In D. Bell and B. Kennedy (eds) *The Cybercultures Reader.* London: Routledge. pp. 77–95.

Robinson, L. and Halle, D. (2002) Digitization, the Internet, and the Arts: eBay, Napster, SAG, and e-Books. *Qualitative Sociology* 25(3): 359–383.

Rodgers, S. and Chen, Q. (2005) Internet Community Group Participation: Psychosocial Benefits for Women with Breast Cancer. *Journal of Computer-Mediated Communication* 10(4): Article 5. Available at http://jcmc.indiana.edu/vol10/issue4/rodgers.html.

Ronai, C. (1994) Narrative Resistance to Deviance: Identity Management among Strip-tease Dancers. *Perspectives on Social Problems* 6: 195–213.

Rose, N. (1992) Governing the Enterprising Self. In P. Heelas and P. Morris (eds) *The Values of Enterprise Culture.* London: Routledge. pp. 141–164.

Rose, N. (2007) Beyond Medicalization. *The Lancet* 369: 700–701.

Sandberg, A. (2001) Morphological Freedom: Why We Not Just Want It, but Need It. Paper given at the TransVision Conference Berlin, 22–24 June.

Sandvik H. (1999) Health Information and interaction on the internet: a survey of female urinary incontinence. *British Medical Journal* 319:29–32.

Sandywell, B. (2006) Monsters in Cyberspace: Cyberphobia and Cultural Panic in the Information Age. *Information, Communication and Society* 9: 39–61.

Saukko, P. (2000) Between Voice and Discourse: Quilting Interviews on Anorexia. *Qualitative Inquiry* 6(3): 299–317.

Scaria, V. (2003) Cyber-pharmacies and Emerging Concerns on Marketing Drugs Online. *Online Journal of Health and Allied Science* 2. Available at www.ojhas.org/issue6/2003–2-1.htm.

Schafernak, K. T. (2000) Organ Commerce Revisited. *Kidney International* 58: 901.

Seale, C. (2002) *Media and Health.* London: Sage.

Seale, C. (2003) Health and Media: An Overview. *Sociology of Health and Illness* 25(6): 513–531.

Seale, C. (2005) New Directions for Critical Internet Health Studies: Representing Cancer Experience on the Web. *Sociology of Health and Illness* 27: 515–540.

Seeman, M.V. (1999) E-Psychiatry: The Patient–Psychiatrist Relationship in the Electronic Age. *Canadian Medical Association Journal* 161(9): 1147–1149.

Seid, R. P. (1994) Too Close to the Bone: The Historical Context for Women's Obsession with Slenderness. In P. Fallon, M.A. Katzman and S.C. Wooley (eds) *Feminist Perspectives on Eating Disorders*. London: Guilford Press. pp. 3–17.

Seidell, J. C. (2000) The Current Epidemic of Obesity. In C. Bouchard (ed.) *Physical Activity and Health*. Champaign, IL: Human Kinetics. pp. 21–30.

Shaikh, T. (2007) Dutch Kidney Donor Show 'a Hoax to Highlight Shortage of Organs'. *Independent*, London, 2 June.

Shepperd, S. and Charnock, D. (2000) Against Internet Exceptionalism: There's Nothing Radically Different about Information on the Web. *British Medical Journal* 324(9), 556–557.

Silagy, C. (1999) Introduction to the New Edition: The Post-Cochrane Agenda: Consumers and Evidence. In A. Cochrane (ed.) *Effectiveness and Efficiency: Random Reflections on Health Service.* London: Royal Society of Medicine Press. pp. 1–7.

Silberg, W. M., Lundberg, G. D. and Musacchio, R. A. (1997) Assessing, Controlling, and Assuring the Quality of Medical Information on the Internet: Caveant Lector et Viewor – Let the Reader and Viewer Beware. *JAMA* 277: 1244–1245.

Simpson, C. (2000) Controversies in Breast Cancer Prevention: The Discourse of Risk. In L. Potts (ed.) *Ideologies of Breast* Cancer. New York: St Martin's Press. pp. 131–152.

Smith, M. (ed.) (2005) *Stelarc: The Monograph.* Cambridge, MA: MIT Press.

Smith, A. D. and Manna, D. R. (2004) Exploring the Trust Factor in e-Medicine. *Online Information Review* 28: 346–355.

Sobchack, V. (2006) A Leg to Stand On: Prosthetics, Metaphor, and Materiality. In M. Smith and J. Morra (eds) (2006) *The Prosthetic Impulse: From a Posthuman Present to a Biocultural Future.* Cambridge, MA: MIT Press. pp. 17–41.

Sontag, S. (1990) *Illness as Metaphor and AIDS and its Metaphors.* New York: Anchor Books Doubleday.

Sørenson, K. H. (2004) Cultural Politics of Technology: Combining Critical and Constructive Interventions. *Science, Technology, and Human Values* 29(2): 184–190.

Spielberg, A. (1998) On call and online: Sociohistorical, legal, and ethical implications of e-mail for the patient–physician relationship. *JAMA* 280(15): 1353–1374.

Spinello, R. A. (2004) Property Rights in Genetic Information. *Ethics and Information Technology* 6: 29–42.

Spoel, P. (2006) Midwifery, Consumerism, and the Ethics of Informed Choice. In P. L. Twohig and V. Kalitzkus (eds) *Bordering Biomedicine: Interdisciplinary Perspectives on Health, Illness, and Disease.* Amsterdam: Rodopi Publications.

Springer, C. (1996) *Electronic Eros: Bodies and Desire in the Postindustrial Age.* London: Athlone Press.

Sproull, L. and Faraj, S. (1995) Atheism, Sex, and Databases: The Net as a Social Technology. In B. Kahin and J. Keller (eds) *Public Access to the Internet.* Cambridge, MA: MIT Press. pp. 62–81.

Spurgeon, D. (2003) US Buyers of Drugs from Canadian Pharmacies Face Prosecution. *British Medical Journal* 326: 618.

Spurlock, M. (2004) *Super Size Me.* USA (film).

Squires, J. (1993) Introduction. In J. Squires (ed.) *Principled Positions: Postmodernism and the Rediscovery of Value.* London: Lawrence and Wishart. pp. 1–16.

Stelarc (1997) From Psycho to Cyber Strategies: Prosthetics, Robotics and Remote Existence. *Cultural Values* 1: 241–249.

Stimson, G. V. (1975) The Message of Psychtropic Drug Ads. *Journal of Communication* 25: 153–160.

Stokals, D. (2000) The Social Ecological Paradigm of Wellness Promotion. In M. S. Jamner and D. Stokals (eds) *Promoting Human Wellness: New Frontiers for Research, Practice, and Policy.* Berkeley: University of California Press. pp. 21–37.

Stryker, S. (2000) Transsexuality: The Postmodern Body and/as Technology. In D. Bell and B. M. Kennedy (eds) *The Cybercultures Reader.* London: Routledge. pp. 588–597.

Suler, J. R. (2001a) The Online Clinical Case Study Group: An E-Mail Model. *CyberPsychology and Behavior* 4(6): 711–722.

Suler, J. R. (2001b) Assessing a Person's Suitability for Online Therapy: The ISMHO Clinical Case Study Group. *CyberPsychology and Behavior* 4(6): 675–679.

Sundén, J. (2001) What Happened to Difference in Cyberspace? The (Re)Turn of the She-Cyborg. *Feminist Media Studies* 1: 215–232.

Tamblyn, C. (1997) Remote Control: The Electronic Transference. In J. Terry and M. Calvert (eds) *Processed Lives: Gender and Technology in Everyday Life.* London: Routledge. pp. 41–46.

Tang, H. and Ng, J. H. K. (2006) Googling for a Diagnosis: Use of Google as a Diagnostic Aid: Internet Based Study. *British Medical Journal* 333: 1143–1145.

Tangen, L. M. and Tjora, A. H. (2002) Surfing for Health: The Internet as Health Information Provider. Paper presented at the BSA Medical Sociology Conference, York, September.

Tan-Torres Edejer, T. (2000) Disseminating Health Information in Developing Countries: The Role of the Internet. *British Medical Journal* 321: 797–800.

Taylor, E. (2002) Totally in Control: The Rise of Pro-Ana/Pro-Mia Websites. Social Issues Research Centre. Available at http://www.sirc.org/articles/totally_in_control.shtml.

Terry, N. P. (1999) Cyber-malpractice: Legal Exposure for Cybermedicine. *Amercian Journal of Law and Medicine* 25: 327.

Thacker, E. (1998) Visible_Human.html/Digital Anatomy and yhe Hyper-texted Body. *CTheory* A060. Available at http://www.ctheory.net/text_file.asp?pick=103.

Thacker, E. (2001) Lacerations: The Visible Human Project, Impossible Anatomies, and the Loss of Corporeal Comprehension. *Culture Machine.* Available at http://culturemachine.tees.ac.uk/Cmach/Backissues/j003/Articles/Thacker/Impossible.htm

Thacker, E. (2003) What Is Biomedia? *Configurations* 11(1): 47–79.

Thompson, J. B. (1995) *The Media and Modernity: A Social Theory of the Media.* Cambridge: Polity Press.

Tiefer, L. (2006) The Viagra Phenomenon. *Sexualities* 9: 273–294.

Treseder, P. (2003) Pro-ana Websites and the Production of Identities, unpublished MSc dissertation. Faculty of Education and Language Studies, The Open University.

Turner, J., Grube, J. and Meyers, J. (2001) Developing an Optimal Match within Online Communities: An Exploration of CMC Support Communities and Traditional Support. *Journal of Communication* 51(2): 231–251.

Turner, L. (2003) Has the President's Council on Bioethics Missed the Boat? *British Medical Journal* 327: 629.

Turner, S. B. (1995) *Medical Power and Social Knowledge.* London: Sage.

Turney, J. (1998) *Frankenstein's Footsteps: Science, Genetics and Popular Culture*. New Haven, CT: Yale University Press.

Urry, J. (2000) *Sociology beyond Societies: Mobilities for the Twenty-First Century*. London: Routledge.

Urwin, R. E., Bennetts, B., Wilcken, B. *et al.* (2002) Anorexia Nervosa (Restrictive Subtype) Is Associated with a Polymorphism in the Novel Norepinephrine Transporter Gene Promoter Polymorphic Region. *Molecular Psychiatry* 7(6): 652–657.

US Department of Health and Human Services (2000) *Healthy People 2010*. Conference edition in two volumes. Washington, DC: US Government Printing Office.

Vares, T. and Braun, V. (2006) Spreading the Word, but What Word Is That? Viagra and Male Sexuality in Popular Culture. *Sexualities* 9: 315–332.

Virilio, P. (1995) Speed and Information: Cyberspace Alarm! *CTheory*, Article 30. Available at www.ctheory.net/text_file?pick=72.

Wachowski, A. and Wachowski, L. (1999) *The Matrix*. Time Warner Entertainment Company, USA (film).

Wakeford, N. (1999) Gender and the Landscapes of Computing in an Internet Cafe. In M. Crang, P. Crang and J. May (eds) *Virtual Geographies: Bodies, Space and Relations*. London and New York: Routledge. pp. 178–201.

Waldby, C. (1997) Revenants: The Visible Human Project and the Digital Uncanny. *Body and Society* 3: 1–16.

Waldby, C. (2000a) *The Visible Human Project: Informatic Bodies and Posthuman Medicine*. London: Routledge.

Waldby, C. (2000b) Virtual Anatomy: From the Body in the Text to the Body on the Screen. *Journal of Medical Humanities* 21(2): 85–107.

Walstrom, M. K. (2000) 'You Know, Who's The Thinnest?': Combating Surveillance and Creating Safety in Coping with Eating Disorders Online. *CyberPsychology and Behavior* 3(5): 761–783.

Ward, J. M. (2003) Online Pharmaceutical Regulation: An Avenue to a Safer World. *Journal of Legal Medicine* 24: 77–107.

Warin, M. (2002) Becoming and Unbecoming: Abject Relations in Anorexia. *Departments of Anthropology and Social Inquiry*. Unpublished doctoral thesis. Adelaide: Adelaide University.

Warin, M. (2003) Miasmatic Calories and Saturating Fats: Fear of Contamination in Anorexia. *Culture, Medicine and Psychiatry* 27: 77–93.

Warin, M. (2004) Primitivising Anorexia: The Irresistible Spectacle of Not Eating. *Australian Journal of Anthropology* 15(1): 95–104.

Webster, A. (2002) Innovative Health Technologies and the Social: Redefining Health, Medicine and the Body. *Current Sociology* 50(3): 443–457.

Weisgerber, C. (2004) Turning to the Internet for Help on Sensitive Medical Problems: A Qualitative Study of the Construction of a Sleep Disorder through Online Interaction. *Information, Communication and Society* 7(4): 554–574.

Weisbord, S. D., Soule, J. B. and Kimmel, P. L. (1997) Poison On Line: Acute Renal Failure Caused by Oil of Wormwood Purchased through the Internet. *New England Journal of Medicine* 337: 825.

Weltao, L. (2007) Internet Users to Log In at World No. 1. *China Daily*.

White, D. (1995) Divide and Multiply: Culture and Politics in the New Medical Order. In P. Komesaroff (ed.) *Troubled Bodies: Critical Perspectives on Postmodernism, Medical Ethics and the Body*. Durham, NC: Duke University Press. pp. 20–37.

Widman, L. E. and Tong, D. A. (1997) Requests for Medical Advice from Patients and Families to Health Care Providers Who Publish on the World Wide Web. *Archives of Internal Medicine* 157(2): 209–212.

Wikipedia (2007, May 27) Web 2.0. Online: http://en.wikipedia.org/wiki/web_2 (accessed 22 April 2007).

Willow, H. (2002) Anorexic Pride Sites Censored! *Hollywood Investigator.* Available at http://www.hollywoodinvestigator.com/2002/anorexic.htm.

Wilson, P. (2002) How to Find the Good and Avoid the Bad or Ugly: A Short Guide to Tools for Rating Quality of Health Information on the Internet. *British Medical Journal* 324: 598–602.

Winker, M. A., Flanagin, A., Chi-Lum, B. *et al.* (2000) Guidelines for Medical and Health Information Sites on the Internet: Principles Governing AMA Web Sites. *JAMA* 283: 1600–1606.

Winzelberg (1997) The Analysis of an Electronic Support group for individuals with eating disorders. *Computers in Human Behaviour* 13(3): 393–407.

Woodward, K. (1999 (originally 1994)) From Virtual Cyborgs to Biological Time Bombs: Technocriticism and the Material Body. In J. Wolmark (ed.) *Cybersexualities: A Reader on Feminist Theory, Cyborgs and Cyberspace.* Edinburgh: Edinburgh University Press. pp. 280–294.

World Health Organization (1998) Obesity, Preventing and Managing the Global Epidemic. Geneva: Report of a WHO Consultation on Obesity.

Worotynec, Z. S. (2000) The Good, The Bad and the Ugly: LISTSERV as Support. *CyberPsychology and Behavior* 3(5): 797–810.

Wright, A. (1999) Partial Bodies: Re-establishing Boundaries, Medical and Virtual. In Cutting Edge: The Women's Research Group (ed.) *Desire by Design: Body, Territories, and New Technologies.* London: I. B. Tauris.

Wright, K. (2000) Perceptions of On-Line Support Providers: An Examination of Perceived Homophily, Source Credibility, Communication and Social Support within On-Line Support Groups. *Communication Quarterly* 48: 44–59.

Wright, K.B. and Bell, S.B. (2003) Health-Related Support Groups on the Internet: Linking Empirical Findings to Social Support and Computer-Mediated Communication Theory. *Journal of Health Psychology* 8(1): 39–54.

Wright, J., and Harwood, V (forthcoming) Governing Bodies: Biopolitics and the 'obesity epidemic', Routledge: London.

Wyatt, S., Henwood, F., Miller, N. and Senker, P. (eds) (2000) *Technology and In/Equality: Questioning the Information Society.* London: Routledge.

Wyatt, S., Henwood, F. and Hart, A. (2005) The Digital Divide, Health Information and Everyday Life. *New Media and Society* 7: 199–218.

Yaskowich, K. M. and Stam, H. J. (2003) Cancer Narratives and the Cancer Support Group. *Journal of Health Psychology* 8(6): 720–737.

Zhai, P. (1997) *Get Real: A Philosophical Adventure in Virtual Reality.* Lanham, MD: Rowman and Littlefield.

Ziebland, S., Chapple, A., Dumelow, C., Evans, J., Prinjha, S. and Rozmovits, L. (2004) How the Internet Affects Patients' Experience of Cancer: A Qualitative Study. *British Medical Journal* 328: 564.

Žižek, S. (2004) *Organs without Bodies: On Deleuze and Consequences.* London: Routledge.

Zola, I. K. (1972) Medicine as an Institution of Social Control. *Sociological Review* 20, 487–503.

Zola, I. K. (1978) Medicine as an Institution of Social Control. In J. Ebrenreich (ed.) *The Cultural Crisis of Modern Medicine.* New York: Monthly Review Press. pp. 80–100.

Zola, I. K. (1998) Medicine as an Institute of Social Control. In L. Mackay, K. Soohill and K. Melia (eds) *Classic Texts in Health Care.* Oxford: Butterworth Heinnemann.

Zylinska, J. (2005) *The Ethics of Cultural Studies.* London: Continuum.

Index